Dubious Equalities and Embodied Differences

Explorations in Bioethics and the Medical Humanities

Series Editor: James Lindemann Nelson

This series aims to include the most theoretically sophisticated, challenging, and original work being produced in the areas of bioethics, literature and medicine, law and medicine, philosophy of medicine, and history of medicine. *Explorations in Bioethics and the Medical Humanities* also features authoritative contributions to educational contexts and to public discourse on the meaning of health and health care in contemporary culture and on the difficult questions concerning the best directions for biomedicine to take in the future.

Dubious Equalities and Embodied Differences

Cultural Studies on Cosmetic Surgery

Kathy Davis

ROWMAN & LITTLEFIELD PUBLISHERS, INC.
Lanham • Boulder • New York • Oxford

ROWMAN & LITTLEFIELD PUBLISHERS, INC.

Published in the United States of America
by Rowman & Littlefield Publishers, Inc.
A Member of the Rowman & Littlefield Publishing Group
4720 Boston Way, Lanham, Maryland 20706
www.rowmanlittlefield.com

PO Box 317
Oxford
OX2 9RU, UK

British Library Cataloguing in Publication Information Available

Library of Congress Cataloging-in-Publication Data
Davis, Kathy, 1949–
    Dubious equalities and embodied differences : cultural studies on
cosmetic surgery / Kathy Davis.
        p. cm.—(Explorations in bioethics and the medical humanities)
    Includes bibliographical references and index.
    ISBN 0-7425-1420-X (hbk. : alk. paper)—ISBN 0-7425-1421-8 (pbk. : alk.
paper)
        1. Surgery, Plastic—Social aspects. I. Title. II. Series.

    RD119.D3848 2003
    617.9'5—dc21   2002154580

Printed in the United States of America

⊚™ The paper used in this publication meets the minimum requirements of American
National Standard for Information Sciences—Permanence of Paper for Printed Library
Materials, ANSI/NISO Z39.48-1992.

Contents

Acknowledgments

This book was not a planned project, conceived and implemented as book. It is the product of my ongoing fascination with cosmetic surgery as cultural phenomenon and my seeming inability to prevent myself from jumping into the fray when I encounter some new development that puzzles, fascinates, or horrifies me. Having already written one book on cosmetic surgery, I thought I was finished with the subject. As the reader will see, I was not.

The book was written over a period of several years and involved my taking on new topics as they caught my fancy, each time with a sense of "I just have to get this one last thing off my chest." Part of what kept me on track and helped consolidate my thinking throughout this period of allowing my passions to guide me was my being fortunate enough to participate in two projects devoted to understanding the ethical aspects of cosmetic surgery.

The first was the Enhancement Project at the Hastings Center, which ran under the able leadership of Erik Parens from 1995 through 1997 and brought together a group of philosophers, physicians, psychologists, sociologists, theologians, and legal scholars to talk about the ethics of technologies for enhancing human appearance and capacities. I profited enormously from these discussions, which were both thought provoking and open enough to allow room for friendly disagreement.

The second project, "Beauty and the Doctor: Moral Issues in Health Care with Regard to Appearance," was inspired by the first and took place on the other side of the Atlantic. Funded by the European Union, it was conceived and organized by a group of bioethicists, primarily from the University of Rotterdam—Inez de Beaufort, Ineke Bolt, Medard Hilhorst, and Henri Wijsbek—and met from 1998 until 2001. I presented several of the chapters from this book in their most rudimentary form during this project and experienced our meetings as the closest thing I have to an "intellectual home." I would like to thank all of the participants for their constructive, challenging, and often entertaining reactions.

Many of the chapters emerged during conversations or public lectures where I was asked to speak about cosmetic surgery. Responses from friends, colleagues, or audiences often provided the impetus for a new chapter. I have thanked these people at the beginning of each chapter, but there are three to whom I owe a special debt:

Dubravka Zarkov was not only the first person to suggest that all of this "might be a book," but she also provided many critical observations, which helped me to sharpen my arguments.

Anna Aalten helped me untangle more theoretical knots than bear thinking about and kept me sane with American movies, bagels, and a much-needed weekend in the country.

Willem de Haan read every chapter several times and—often miraculously—seemed to know not only where the problem lay, but also how to fix it. I am deeply thankful that he is the person I—hopefully—will be growing old with and will have around for the next book as well.

Parts of this book have appeared in the following earlier versions.

Chapter 1, "Cosmetic Surgery in a Different Voice," from *Women's Studies International Forum* 22, no. 5 (1999): 473–88.

Chapter 2, "Pygmalions in Plastic Surgery," from *Health: An Interdisciplinary Journal for the Social Study of Health, Illness and Medicine* 2, no. 1 (1998): 23–40.

Chapter 3, "'The Rhetoric of Cosmetic Surgery: Luxury or Welfare?" from *Enhancing Human Traits: Ethical and Social Implications*, edited by Erik Parens. Washington, D.C.: Georgetown University Press, 1998.

Chapter 4, "From Objectified Body to Embodied Subject," from *Feminist Social Psychologies: International Perspectives*, edited by Sue Wilkinson. Philadelphia: Open University Press, 1996.

Chapter 6, "'My Body Is My Art:' Cosmetic Surgery as Feminist Utopia?" from *European Journal of Women's Studies* 4, no.1 (1997): 23–38.

Chapter 7, "'A Dubious Equality': Men, Women and Cosmetic Surgery," from *Body & Society* 8, no. 1 (2002): 49–65.

Introduction

Several years ago, I completed a book about women's involvement in cosmetic surgery, *Reshaping the Female Body* (1995). As is often the case after putting so much time and energy into a subject, I was more than ready to move on to a new topic. However, I soon discovered—and somewhat to my dismay—that the subject of cosmetic surgery was not to be left behind. For one thing, the field itself is constantly expanding. Even if I had wanted to forget about cosmetic surgery, the media bombards us all with its tireless coverage of the latest and often quite bizarre techniques for reshaping and beautifying the body: "ear lobe tucks," the elimination of frown wrinkles through paralyzing facial muscles with botulism injections, vulva reductions—the list is endless. Overviews abound of available interventions, often using the same imagery, the same diagram of a woman's body with arrows pointing to body parts with the name of the operation and its price, the only difference being the language and currency. Clinics all over the world advertise their services, invariably with the before-and-after picture.[1] Potential targets of the "surgical fix" have expanded, however, from women to include men, "ethnic minorities," or the disabled (for example, leg lengthening for dwarves). And, the atrocity stories have become more dramatic. The surgical exploits of Cher and Michael Jackson, which graced the pages of women's magazines throughout the nineties, seem pale next to the dramatic tale of Lolo Ferrari, the French actress and singer whose eight-pound breast implants may have contributed to her untimely death at age thirty.[2] Cosmetic surgery continues to elicit public controversy—where reconstruction ends and aesthetic surgery begins, who should be allowed to do it and where,[3] or which kinds of interventions should or should not be covered by medical insurance. More recently, debates have extended to

1

more encompassing ethical issues like where to draw the line in altering the "natural" body or whether biotechnologies should be used to solve social or cultural problems.

But it is not just the ongoing attention paid to cosmetic surgery in the media that held my attention. The past decade has marked an enormous upsurge of scholarly interest in the body. Conferences on the body abound, and no annual meeting in the social sciences, cultural studies, or humanities would be complete without at least one session devoted to the body. A whole series of "body" books has emerged, and there is even a journal devoted entirely to the "body." This trend, which has been dubbed the "new body theory," shows no signs of waning (see Davis 1997). Within this interdisciplinary scholarship on the body, cosmetic surgery remains a topic. It touches on theoretically interesting issues concerning identity and embodiment. It provides a perfect illustration of the obsession in Western late modern cultures with the makeability of the body. And, last but not least, it offers the possibility for exploring the political and ethical implications of biotechnological expansion.

Thus, even if I had wanted to forget cosmetic surgery, its ubiquitous presence in scientific and popular discourse would have made that impossible. Nevertheless, the incentive for writing another book on the subject required an extra nudge—and this nudge came with a little help from my friends.

"HAVE YOU SEEN THIS?"

My husband hands me a battered and dog-eared book with old-fashioned typesetting and yellowing pages and, laughing mischievously, says: "I couldn't resist." And, indeed, how could he have? The book had the intriguing title *Doctor Pygmalion: The Autobiography of a Plastic Surgeon*. The frontispiece was a smiling photograph of the author, Maxwell Maltz, looking like a 1940s movie star with wavy hair and bedroom eyes. I discovered that Maltz was one of the pioneers of modern cosmetic surgery, who, having reached the end of his illustrious career, had seen fit to write his autobiography. I was fascinated. I had, of course, ample opportunity in my previous research to talk to plastic surgeons, many of whom—true to the stereotype—were competitive, arrogant, Porsche-driving machos. While the title seemed to express the all-too-familiar hubris and misogyny I had come to expect among cosmetic surgeons, the format—an autobiography—promised a more intimate look, a glimpse behind the professional veneer. Vaguely curious, I began to read about Dr. Pygmalion—and along with it—several other surgeon biographies—leading, ultimately, to the second essay of this book.

My curiosity aroused, I soon discovered other pioneers, among whom the indomitable Madame Noël—the first (and one of the few) women plastic surgeons. She had not only been instrumental in developing the "face-lift," but had been a famous feminist as well. At this point, I was beginning to enjoy following up interesting leads. I discovered that Noël had written one of the first handbooks on cosmetic surgery and, after searching the libraries in the Netherlands, discovered an ancient copy of a German translation (the original had been in French) in the library of the University of Leyden. The librarian was clearly surprised that anyone could be interested in this particular book (it hadn't been checked out for forty years), but he was kind enough to send it to me. One look and I couldn't put it down. I read it in one sitting, entranced at how completely different this text was from anything I had encountered in the world of medicine. This encounter led to the first essay of this book in which I explore the gendered underpinnings of cosmetic surgery from the vantage point of a "different voice."

These two excursions might have remained just that—brief and somewhat idiosyncratic forays into the beginnings of modern cosmetic surgery. However, while I was snooping around in archives, my book *Reshaping the Female Body* was generating some controversy. I was frequently asked to provide the feminist perspective on cosmetic surgery on radio and television programs, usually together with a plastic surgeon and a representative of the "beauty industry." In addition to the latest "nip and tuck" or the inevitable question about whether I thought men were in danger of becoming the new victims of the Beauty Myth, I was asked to comment on the performance artist Orlan, whose art involved having her face surgically reconstructed in front of the video camera. Not only did journalists wonder what made cosmetic surgery as art different from "ordinary" cosmetic surgery, but feminist colleagues, admiring Orlan's postmodern identity manipulations, saw similarities between our theoretical projects.

Gradually, I found myself getting drawn into discussions about the meaning of cosmetic surgery in contemporary cultural life: what did Orlan's project imply about women's agency, why were men any different than women when it came to beauty, or what was wrong with having surgery to eliminate an "ethnic" nose? These discussions raised theoretical and normative issues, which were controversial enough for me to respond, often motivated by the desire to "set the record straight." Several of the essays in this book are the result of my attempts to tackle my theoretical or moral unease about different manifestations of cosmetic surgery.

And, finally, *Reshaping the Female Body* evoked controversy among feminist scholars. It had been written against the backdrop of the long-standing feminist critique of the beauty system that views cosmetic surgery as a particularly reprehensible beauty practice that is not only risky to women's health but sustains cultural notions of feminine inferiority (Bartky 1990; Young 1990b; Morgan 1991; Bordo 1993). After listening to women's stories about their suffering with their appearance as well as their struggles to over-come this suffering, however, I had become dissatisfied with a critique of cosmetic surgery as a beauty practice—a critique that allowed even well-intentioned feminists to trivialize women's reasons for having surgery or to reduce them to ideological mystification. Women's surgical stories told a different tale. They showed how cosmetic surgery can be a less than satisfactory way to redress a situation that is too painful to endure, both problem and solution, all in one. As a result of my inquiry, cosmetic surgery took on the shape of a dilemma that required nothing less than a balancing act between a critique of the technologies, practices, and discourses that define women's bodies as deficient and in need of change and a sociological understanding of why women might view cosmetic surgery as their best—and, in some cases—only option for alleviating unbearable suffering. My approach resonated with—and, in some cases encouraged—other feminist scholars to explore women's agency in other—similarly unlikely—practices ranging from makeup use (Dellinger and Williams 1997), ballet (Aalten 1997), hormone replacement therapy (Klinge 1997), pornography (Chancer 1998), beauty pageants (Banet-Weiser 1999), and transsexuality (Phibbs 2001) to hymen reconstructions (Saharso 2002). They also engaged in similar feminist "balancing acts" in which they combined a critical analysis of potentially problematic body practices with a respectful reading of women's experiences and reasons for doing them. Other feminist scholars were concerned about my focus on agency, however, labeling it theoretically misguided and politically dangerous (Bordo 1993 and 1997). Their criticisms of my work provided a welcome opportunity to elaborate some of the issues, which had not been sufficiently addressed in my book and which, indirectly, led to this new book.

This book is based on a series of essays, which have been written since the publication of *Reshaping the Female Body*, often in response to new developments in the field of cosmetic surgery. Taken together, they provide a critical interrogation of the process by which cosmetic surgery has been taken up into Western cultures of late modernity. I draw upon a wide range of cultural manifestations of the current preoccupation with cosmetic surgery, taking my examples from different sources: the media, performance art, biographies of well-known surgeons, surgical stories from patients, public debates, and medical texts. Some of the texts are historical—for example, (auto)biographies of pioneers in cosmetic surgery or early handbooks on cosmetic surgery. Other texts are contemporary—for example, media coverage of new interventions like penile augmentations, medical debates about the financial and ethical implications of cosmetic surgery, or representations of cosmetic surgery as "body art." It has not been my intention to provide typical cases—although some are certainly representative and will be familiar to most readers. Many of my cases have been selected precisely because they seem, at first glance, to be atypical as, for example, a feminist cosmetic surgeon or the artist Orlan who uses cosmetic surgery as an art form.

The underlying theme of the book concerns the tension between equality ("each of us has the right to the body he or she desires") and differences in embodiment as an integral and unavoidable part of the human condition. This tension is played out in the discourses and practices of cosmetic surgery in medicine, in personal stories, in public debates, and in popular culture. Notions of equality and discourse inform medical discourse about what constitutes "normal" or desirable appearance as well as what constitutes appropriate surgical intervention. They are integral to how individuals make sense of their suffering with their appearance and how they justify their decisions to have their bodies altered surgically. They shape—explicitly or implicitly— contemporary debates about the politics and ethics of cosmetic surgery. They also find expression in representations of cosmetic surgery in popular culture, the media, and the arts.

DISCOURSES OF EQUALITY
AND EMBODIED DIFFERENCES

Cosmetic surgery is predicated upon definitions of physical normality. It was developed to alleviate deviations in normal appearance, and, indeed, the recent "revolution" in cosmetic surgery attests to plastic surgeons' increasing authority to distinguish between normal and abnormal bodies. In Western culture, the white, propertied male has enjoyed the normative position against which all others—women, the working classes, or the ethnically marginalized—are measured and found wanting. It is hardly surprising that women have been the particular targets of cosmetic surgery. Cosmetic surgery was not specifically intended as an intervention in femininity. However, in a sexist, racist, or class society, certain groups (women, the ethnically marginalized, elderly people, homosexuals, disabled or fat people) are defined as "ugly, fearful or loathsome" through a process that Iris Marion Young (1990a) refers to as the "aesthetic scaling of bodies" (123–24). Individuals who represent groups falling outside white, Western, middle-class norms are defined through their bodily characteristics and constructed as different, as "Other." They find themselves under pressure to at least appear "normal" and, consequently, may be prepared to go to extreme lengths to achieve a normal-looking body. In a culture where feminine beauty is idealized, the "aesthetic scaling of bodies" specifically structures the dynamics of gender oppression, rendering ordinary-looking women ugly and deficient and trapping them into the hopeless race for a perfect body. Or, as Bernice Hausman (1995) somewhat ironically notes: "If women can't be normal because of their sex, they might as well be perfect" (65).

In *Reshaping the Female Body*, I showed how the categories of "normality" and "abnormality" are drawn upon in both medical discourse on cosmetic surgery—how cosmetic surgeons justify their professional practice, setting the parameters for debates about professional, technical, and ethical implications of cosmetic surgery—and in individual's accounts of their surgical experiences—how they made sense of their suffering with their appearance or justified their decisions to have their bodies altered surgically. Cosmetic surgery becomes a legitimate reaction to the desire to appear normal ("just like everyone else"). Surgeons have had to defend cosmetic surgery against accusations of quackery (operating on healthy bodies), triviality (pampering their patient's vanity), and capriciousness (cosmetic surgery as luxury). To this end, they have argued that cosmetic surgery is necessary in a culture where appearance is important to a person's happiness and well-being; it is a requirement for a patient's welfare (see chapter 3).

Since writing the book, however, cosmetic surgery has not only been taken up increasingly by the media and in popular culture. Cultural discourses about bodies and embodiment have shifted, altering the way cosmetic surgery is represented as well. Difference has become a "commodity," with none of the negative associations with which "abnormality" is imbued. Differences in color, sex and sexuality, or nation are celebrated (Lury 2000). Multiculturalism is the ostensible ideal in morphed images like the SimEve gracing the cover of *Time* magazine (Haraway 1997). "Race" or "sex," once markers of inequality, have now become a matter of stylistic choice, something that can be mixed and matched like putting on different outfits. The body is simply a vehicle for recognizing our individual desires and projects. In short, the Benetton ideal reigns supreme.

In this cultural context, cosmetic surgery is increasingly presented as neutral technology, ideally suited to altering the body in accordance with an individual's personal preferences. This can include enhancing femininity or eradicating physical features associated with ethnicity or "race." After all, why are pectoral implants on a man any different than silicone implants for a woman? And, what is the difference between dreadlocks on a white teenager and the widespread practice of hair straightening among Afro-American women (Rooks 1996; Banks 2000)? The discourse of "we are all different," along with individual choice and neutral technology, seems to have taken cosmetic surgery out of the "old" discourse of normality and abnormality and allowed it to transcend such categories altogether. Cosmetic surgery promises a different body, but this time, a body that has nothing to do with normative constraints associated with gender or "race" or nationality. Indeed, it seems to promise a society where problematic differences—differences that are associated with structured or systematic social inequalities—have been smoothed out, "homogenized," or eliminated altogether. Once invisible, they will ostensibly cease to exist. Or, as Michael Jackson, one of the most vocal recipients of cosmetic surgery has noted, "Black or white? I'm tired of being a color" (see chapter 5).

The celebration of individuality and erasure of systematic embodied difference seems to suggest a desirable kind of equality (we are all individuals, the same no matter how we look or what the particular circumstances of our lives are). This focus on equality is, however, not without problems, as various feminist cultural critics have convincingly demonstrated.[4] Applied to current cultural phenomenon of cosmetic surgery, I see, in particular, three problems with equality discourse.

The first problem is that equality discourse downplays the significance of cosmetic surgery, trivializing its dangers and transforming it into a neutral technology that can be deployed by any individual in the interests of his or her personal "identity project." As long as cosmetic surgery was viewed as a solution for "abnormal" appearance (however spurious that category has been in the past), it could be treated as an exceptional solution for an exceptional problem. However, if all individuals are "equally" different, then anyone can be a potential candidate for surgical intervention. Cosmetic surgery—like any other consumer good—is a matter of personal preference and the means to afford it. Thus, the threshold to the surgeon's office is lowered, making cosmetic surgery an option for individuals who might not have considered it before.

The second problem with equality discourse is that it deflects attention from structural inequalities based on gender, ethnicity, nationality, age, or other categories of difference. It ignores specific histories and current conditions of inequality, which give body practices different meanings. Cher's decision to have her belly button tucked or her bottom rib removed is not the same as an Asian American teenager choosing to have her eyes Westernized. Treating these interventions as commensurate—both a matter of individual choice, both equally responsive to the current beauty ideals—depoliticizes cosmetic surgery. It discounts the universality of white, Western norms of appearance, which shape individuals' perceptions of what they consider to be desirable appearance as well as the kinds of interventions that are deemed acceptable. Not every body will do; nor are all differences the same in Western culture. Eyes are rarely made to look more "oriental," any more than noses are made to look more "Jewish." Thus, one ideal—a white, Western model—becomes the norm to which everyone, explicitly or implicitly, aspires. Cosmetic surgery becomes decontextualized and depoliticized when changes in appearance are seen has having the same cultural meaning and the same political (or normative) valence. In effect, this means that cosmetic surgery has *no* cultural meaning and *no* [her italics] political valence (Bordo 1993, 253).

The third problem with equality discourse is that it ignores the individual's interactions with her or his material, fleshy body and, through this body, with the outside world. Bodies are not like pieces of clothing, to be donned or taken off at will. Individuals have specific histories of suffering with their bodies, born of their interactions with others. Their embodiment takes shape within specific cultural constraints, which require ongoing negotiation. When the media proclaims that men have become the "new" victims of the beauty craze (see chapter 7), women's long-standing tradition of suffering "for the sake of beauty" is not only downplayed, but men's specific experiences with *their* bodies in the context of culturally specific discourses and practices of masculinity are ignored as well. Equality discourse erases the specificity, which allows us to understand the lived experience of embodiment within concrete historical, social, and cultural contexts.

In short, equality discourse seems to stand in the way of a critical understanding of cosmetic surgery precisely because it ignores embodied difference. However, my uneasiness is not limited to how cosmetic surgery is represented in the media and popular culture. Some of the problems of this discourse may also be found in more scholarly treatises on the body and contemporary beauty culture.

THEORIZING BODY CULTURE

The contemporary body culture has been the subject of considerable theorizing, particularly among feminists (see Davis 1997). They have shown how beauty practices are integral to the construction of femininity in a gendered social order. Originally, women were regarded as victims of an oppressive "beauty system" that included the media, the cosmetics industry, cultural beauty ideals, and, last but not least, cosmetic surgery. Under the influence of post-structuralist theory—in particular, Foucault—more sophisticated frameworks have gradually been developed to explore the insidious and ambivalent ways that women's bodies are disciplined through beauty practices and discourses (Bartky 1990; Bordo 1993). Femininity has come to be regarded less as a cultural script than a series of performances, ongoing in process and always subject to subversion or "gender trouble" (Butler 1990 and 1993). Simplified notions of power that relegated women to the role of duped victim of a uniformly oppressive "beauty system" have been elaborated to include a concern for women's agency as well as for the complexity and ambivalence of their involvement in beauty practices.

While these shifts in feminist theory have been productive, they have not been without problems. Postmodern body theory has often been a cerebral, esoteric, and—ironically—disembodied activity, which distances us from individuals' everyday embodied experiences and practices. There has been an unmistakable ambivalence toward the material body and a tendency to privilege the body as metaphor. "Experience," once the mainstay of feminist scholarship, has now become an object for deconstruction rather than a starting point for understanding how experience is ongoingly constructed, as "meaning in action" (Young 1990b).[5] The postmodern focus on identity as fragmented, multilayered, and fluctuating has shifted attention from structured categories of difference like gender, "race," and class, while domination and constraint are often downplayed in favor of a concern for individual agency and subversion.

I have taken issue with some of the problems inherent in postmodern feminist scholarship on the body. In an essay with the telling title, "Embodying Theory: Beyond Modernist and Postmodernist Readings of the Body," for example, I criticized theories on the body that ignored the particularities of individuals' experiences and practices as well as the concrete social, cultural, and historical contexts in which they are embedded (Davis 1997, 15). In *Reshaping the Female Body*, I provided a feminist reading of cosmetic surgery that is grounded in the specific histories of suffering of those women who undergo it as well as in a critique of the culture that makes the surgical alteration of bodies seem like a "solution" for their suffering.

Given my own ambivalent relationship to postmodern feminist theory on the body, I was somewhat taken aback to find myself relegated in no uncertain terms to the camp of postmodern feminism by one of its most respected critics—Susan Bordo. Since I not only share many of her criticisms of (postmodern) feminist theory, but have drawn upon her work extensively both in *Reshaping the Female Body* and the present volume, I feel called upon to clarify some of the issues that seem to be at stake in her critique of my work. These issues are, I believe, fundamental to any critical discussion of the cultural significance of cosmetic surgery.

BORDO ON *RESHAPING THE FEMALE BODY*

A philosopher by training, Susan Bordo has provided a penetrating analysis of the current cultural obsession with slenderness, including eating disorders, the fitness craze, and—last but not least—cosmetic surgery. Much of her work entails a critical deconstruction of representations of women's bodies in popular culture (advertisements, television, films). Drawing upon Foucauldian notions of power, she shows how processes of normalization (measuring women's bodies against contemporary ideals of femininity) and homogenization (the containment of disturbing bodily differences) are integral to the contemporary body culture. Even more pernicious, however, is the discourse of choice and the mentality of personal empowerment ("Just Do It!") that permeates popular culture.

In Bordo's view, this discourse is not only employed in the media, or echoed by women who defend their decisions to have their faces "lifted" or their tummies "tucked." It is also employed by postfeminists like Naomi Wolf (1993) or Katie Roiphe (1993), who criticize "old feminists" for viewing women as victims and refusing to respect their choices. However, even their more "moderate, sober, scholarly sisters" who, under the influence of post-structuralist theory, "celebrate" women's agency, are guilty of jumping on the freedom bandwagon (Bordo 1997, 35). It is to this latter brand of feminism, which Bordo calls "agency feminism," that my work on cosmetic surgery belongs.

According to Bordo, I have gone overboard in taking women who have cosmetic surgery at their word (Bordo 1997, 35–36). Just because they claim that cosmetic surgery is their best option under the circumstances, doesn't mean that I should take their words at face value. By directing my attention to individual women's experiences with their bodies and their decisions to have cosmetic surgery in *Reshaping the Female Body*, I have missed the bigger picture. I have not only *denied* the systematic constraints that operate on women and compel them to have their bodies altered surgically, but am guilty of *condoning* cosmetic surgery and the beauty industry as "in fact play(ing) an important role in *empowering* women" [my italics] (Bordo 1997, 35–36).

Bordo (1997) claims that *Reshaping the Female Body* is "dominated" by metaphors of choice and freedom—of women "taking their life into their own hands (35)." Structural constraints like sexism and racism are nothing more than "hurdles to be jumped" or "personal challenges to be overcome (34)." Since the same metaphors of choice and freedom can be found in contemporary advertising campaigns, Bordo concludes that my analysis unwittingly supports the pernicious discourse of individualism and personal empowerment, which is endemic to contemporary Western culture. She does not deny that I—or feminists like me—am aware of the power of cultural images and their contribution to women's viewing their bodies as defective and unacceptable. However, by focusing "*first and foremost* [her italics] on women's agency" and by describing their decisions as a "locus of creativity, power, and self-definition," *Reshaping the Female Body* has failed to give sufficient attention to the systematic constraints that operate on women and compel them to have cosmetic surgery (Bordo 1993, 20; Bordo 1997, 36, 42). A critical cultural analysis of cosmetic surgery would entail putting the systematic and institutional features of the beauty culture at the forefront of the analysis rather than exploring and giving credence to individual women's experiences and choices.

While Bordo has been critical herself of early feminist portrayals of power as too simplistic, she, nevertheless, chastises me for unfairly accusing "old feminists" (her term) of "wallowing in the victim state" and refusing to "honor and respect" the choices women make (Bordo 1997, 35–36). In this respect, I am no better than Naomi Wolf and Katie Roiphe. She objects to my view that feminist scholarship "needs to be corrected," arguing that I have thereby played into the recent feminist backlash that defames any feminist analysis that focuses on "unpopular" structural inequalities as "old-fashioned," unnecessary, or too politically correct.

Bordo assumes that one of the primary problems of contemporary culture is that its workings are not obvious to most of us. In fact, we are continually "tricked" by false promises of individual freedom, choice, and the possibility of controlling our lives by manipulating our bodies. It is difficult for most of us to see structures of inequality based on sexism or racism, when they are constantly being obscured by discourses of individualism and the primacy of "mind" over "matter." Bordo, therefore, sees it as her task to become a "diagnostician" of culture. She situates herself as someone who must "excavate and explore" the "hidden and unquestioned aspects" of Western culture that treat women and other marginalized individuals as abhorrent or inferior and deny systematic structures of domination under the guise of individual freedom (Bordo 1997, 174). In her view, any cultural analysis worth its salt has to provide a "picture of the landscape" and not just "individual snapshots" (43).

In actual fact, I suspect that Bordo and I have rather similar theoretical and normative agendas. However, her criticisms also suggest that there are differences in how we approach cultural phenomena like cosmetic surgery. In particular, we differ in our use of "agency" and our conception of what a feminist cultural critique should entail. As both are central to understanding the cultural significance of cosmetic surgery and, consequently, to the present inquiry, I will provide a brief rejoinder.[6]

THE PROBLEM OF AGENCY

"Agency" as a sociological concept plays a central role in my inquiry into women's involvement in cosmetic surgery. I drew upon agency to help me understand how women could view cosmetic surgery—a costly, painful, dangerous, and demeaning practice—as their best and—in some cases—only option under the circumstances. Bordo conflates my use of "agency" with the discourses of "choice" and "freedom" that she finds in the media and in popular culture. "Agency" as a term is rarely found in the media, however, let alone in advertising jargon. It is a sociological concept and refers to the active participation of individuals in the constitution of social life. It does not represent "free choice," although individuals generally have some degree of freedom in their actions in the sense of, in most cases, being able to act otherwise. Individual agency is always situated in relations of power, which provide the conditions of enablement and constraint under which all social action takes place. There is no "free space" where individuals exercise "choice" in any absolute sense of the word. "Choices" are always messy affairs, rarely undertaken with perfect knowledge of circumstances, let alone certain or predictable outcomes.

The relationship between agency and structure has been the subject of one of the most long-standing and important debates within social sciences during the past century.[7] What is at stake in the sociological use of agency is how to understand the ways that social action and social structures are mutually constitutive and sustaining without falling into the twin traps of methodological individualism, on the one hand, and structural determinism, on the other. Agency is invariably linked to social structures and yet never entirely reducible to them. It is always multilayered, involving a complicated mix of intentionality, practical knowledge, and unconscious motives.

It is in this context that my focus on women's agency (including my use of another sociological notion, "cultural dope") should be seen—as a needed corrective of overly deterministic accounts of social action, which I perceived in some feminist scholarship on women's involvement in the "beauty system." It was hardly my intention to "accuse" or "blame" feminists, as Bordo (1997, 35) suggests. Given the pervasiveness of the constraints upon women to meet the cultural ideals of feminine appearance, it almost goes without saying that feminists will be inclined to view women who have cosmetic surgery— the most dramatic beauty practice of all—as victims of ideological manipulation. This was also my initial response as feminist—something I explained at length in my introduction of *Reshaping the Female Body* (Davis 1995, 1–5). However, it was a response that also seemed too easy. As Giddens (1976), one of the leading social theorists of agency, has pointed out: "every competent actor has a wide-ranging, but intimate and subtle, knowledge of the society of which he or she is a member" (73). By underlining this knowledgeability, social action does not suddenly become a matter of "doing one's own thing." But neither can it be reduced to a simple knee-jerk reflex of social forces, imposed upon unwitting or deluded individuals. A focus on agency opens the door to a sociological exploration of how people draw upon their knowledge of themselves and their circumstances as they negotiate their everyday lives.

It was in this sense—analogous to Giddens[8]—that I tried to avoid what would have been relatively easy for me, as feminist, to do—namely, to treat women as deluded by the false promises of the feminine beauty system, as "cultural dopes." Instead I took a more analytic stance and tried to make sense of what—at least initially—did not make sense to me. Against my own inclination to view women who have cosmetic surgery as "cultural dopes," I positioned them as "competent actors" with an "intimate and subtle knowledge of society," including the dominant discourses and practices of feminine beauty. This approach enabled me to understand what I had not been able to understand before—namely, why, given their specific experiences with their bodies and the possibilities available to them for alleviating their suffering, cosmetic surgery could be an action of choice, solution and problem, empowering and disempowering, all at once.[9]

However, even if Bordo and I were to agree that our difference of opinion on the problem of "agency" is theoretical or the result of our disciplinary backgrounds, I believe that more is at stake in her critique of my work than agency. The question of whether a consideration of individual women's stories is relevant for a feminist cultural critique of cosmetic surgery and, more generally, what a cultural critique of ethically or politically problematic practices like cosmetic surgery should entail may be even more salient.

CULTURAL CRITIQUE

In *Reshaping the Female Body,* I chose to explore what Bordo has called "individual snapshots"—that is, women's stories of suffering and their attempts to overcome their suffering through cosmetic surgery—because these stories tend to get lost in debates about the ethical and political implications of cosmetic surgery. This is hardly a new research strategy and as most feminist scholars would agree, women's voices have often required some "retrieval" as they often tend to get lost between the cracks. Bordo has herself admitted that it was a good thing to "listen to those women."[10] However, the problems begin when I not only "listen" to what they say, but treat what they have to say as consequential for a critical feminist perspective on cosmetic surgery.

Based on "these women's" accounts, I came to appreciate that women often have "good"—that is, credible and justifiable—reasons for wanting to have cosmetic surgery. This does not mean that I "condone" the practice, let alone the cultural norms that make women hate their bodies and long to have them altered. Indeed—I discovered that most of the women I spoke with don't condone cosmetic surgery either, but are, typically, highly critical of it, arguing that it is only defensible in specific cases (notably, their own) to relieve suffering that has passed a point of what a person should have to endure.

But taking women at their word is not simply a matter of "honoring their choices." It is precisely my concern about the continued popularity of cosmetic surgery—even in the face of increased media coverage of the risks and drawbacks—that made it seem imperative for me to understand why individual women were so determined to undertake it. Cosmetic surgery is not just popular; it is also controversial. Recipients struggle with the side effects and dangers of the surgery, welfare bureaucrats and insurance companies worry about the costs, and even surgeons express objections about whether surgery should be performed on otherwise healthy bodies just "for looks." While these concerns do not necessarily result in a refusal of the practice, the hesitations, which participants express and which are embedded in public debates about cosmetic surgery, provide insight into what makes cosmetic surgery not only desirable, but also problematic. Looking at the ambivalences that are already present can not only help us understand what is at stake with cosmetic surgery; it can enable us to see how, under different circumstances, another course of action might have been possible.

Unlike Bordo, I do not see myself as an "excavator" of hidden truths. The assumption that I could adopt the privileged position of someone who unearths hitherto unknown truths about culture presents some rather obvious difficulties. On what ground am I to discover the hidden truth of the culture to which I belong, while others are doomed to muddle along, blinded by their culture and, unlike me, unable to make sense of it? But even if I were able to justify taking such a privileged position, my conception of what constitutes critical cultural analysis differs from Bordo's.

In *Reshaping the Female Body*, I described myself as engaged in a "feminist balancing act"—balancing on a "razor's edge":

> between a feminist critique of the cosmetic surgery craze (along with the ideologies of feminine inferiority which sustain it) and an equally feminist desire to treat women as agents who negotiate their bodies and their lives within the cultural and structural constraints of a gendered social order. This has meant exploring cosmetic surgery as one of the most pernicious expressions of the Western beauty culture without relegating women who have it to the position of "cultural dope." It has involved understanding how cosmetic surgery might be the best possible course of action for a particular woman, while, at the same time, problematizing the situational constraints which make cosmetic surgery an option. (Davis 1995, 5)

In order to engage in this balancing act, I had to draw upon my own "intimate and subtle knowledge of society." My membership in the very culture I was criticizing was an indispensable resource that helped me to recognize the dilemmas confronting women who have cosmetic surgery as well as the cultural discourses they used to explain, criticize, but also justify or defend the practice. If I had anything special to offer as a critic, it was not the truth, let alone a higher moral ground. Rather I demonstrated a willingness to entertain the unease and—at times—outright discomfort—which cosmetic surgery evokes, particularly among feminists, and to do so long enough to unravel what might be at stake in some of its dilemmas.

Cosmetic surgery evokes deep-seated apprehension and ambivalence. In the present inquiry, I have, once again, gravitated toward features of cosmetic surgery as cultural phenomenon, which are puzzling, troubling, or, quite simply, don't make sense to me, and used them as an occasion for further exploration. I have engaged with certain points of view, precisely because they expressed sentiments that were different and sometimes even antithetical to my own. While this often made me uncomfortable, it also provided an opportunity to understand aspects of "our" cultural obsession with the makeability of the body that might otherwise have been unavailable to me. But, more important, it allowed me to keep a discussion open in what the philosopher Paul Ricoeur (1999) in his ethics of conflict has called "reasonable disagreement."[11] I concluded *Reshaping the Female Body* with the line: "as feminist critics of cosmetic surgery, we cannot afford the comfort of the 'correct line.'" Given the visibility and impact of cosmetic surgery in our contemporary cultural landscape, I believe that—if anything—it is even more essential as cultural critics to find ways to keep the discussion about cosmetic surgery open, so that we can explore what makes it both popular and problematic.

ABOUT THIS BOOK

This book begins with a brief foray into the history of cosmetic surgery. Taking one of the pioneers as a case in point, I show how the inventor of the all-too-familiar "face-lift" could also be a committed feminist. Given the role cosmetic surgery—and, more generally, the feminine beauty system—plays in disciplining and denigrating women's bodies, a feminist cosmetic surgeon seemed a highly unlikely combination. However, based on an analysis of her life and her work, I show how it is possible to do cosmetic surgery "in a different voice." At the same time, I open my analysis of the gendered underpinnings of the profession and practice of cosmetic surgery.

The next chapter provides a contrasting case. Drawing upon a popular autobiography of another pioneer of the profession, I show how masculinity and cosmetic surgery are intertwined. I use this autobiography—with the telling title of *Doctor Pygmalion*—as a resource for understanding the discourses that shaped—and continue to shape—the profession of plastic surgery. By analyzing the textual practices, which the author employs to construct his life as the idealized story of a plastic surgeon, the professional ideology of plastic surgery as well as the construction of masculinity in its professionalized form is explored.

Since the early days of cosmetic surgery, medical interventions in the human body have burgeoned. From open-heart surgery to organ transplants to gene therapy, the possibilities for technological enhancement seem almost unlimited. While these interventions are supposed to prolong life, improve health, and promote well-being, in practice, they are often dangerous, expensive, and morally problematic. In the third chapter, I explore some of the problems that emerge to justify cosmetic surgery, arguably one of the most controversial of the new biotechnologies. To make my case, I draw upon public debates in the Netherlands where—in contrast to the United States and other Western European nations—cosmetic surgery was covered by National Health and defended as "welfare surgery." Based on this—admittedly— exceptional case, I will discuss some of the limitations of a moral rhetoric based on equality, universality, and distributive justice, and with the help of contemporary feminist ethics, put forth an approach to cosmetic surgery that takes a politics of difference, particularity, and need interpretation as its normative starting point.

Having looked at the public face of cosmetic surgery, in chapter 4 I turn to the personal stories that the recipients of cosmetic surgery tell. Based on the biographical analysis of surgical narratives, I show how they make sense of their problematic relationship to their bodies and through their bodies to the world around them. Taking issue with psychological, sociological, and feminist scholarship on women's preoccupation with appearance, I show how the desire for cosmetic surgery may be more about wanting to be ordinary ("just like everyone else") than being beautiful. Drawing upon a narrative perspective on identity, I propose that cosmetic surgery be regarded as an occasion for renegotiating one's identity and, paradoxically, for becoming an embodied subject rather than "just a body."

Cosmetic surgery is not just a means toward the "enhancement" of appearance. Traditionally, it has entailed the eradication of markers of "difference"— that is, different from dominant or more desirable ethnic groups. In chapter 5, I raise the question of how "ethnic cosmetic surgery" (presented as a "new" branch of cosmetic surgery) is different from other types of cosmetic surgery, including surgery for enhancing femininity. Drawing upon on analysis of medical texts as well as the case of Michael Jackson, I show why an intersectional perspective is essential for making sense of the racialized underpinnings of cosmetic surgery as well as the relative ease or unease that cosmetic surgery in its different manifestations evokes.

At first glance, cosmetic surgery seems to represent the epitome of the colonization and victimization of women through their bodies. In recent years, however, postmodern feminist scholars have begun to explore the possibilities of the technologized female body as a site for feminist action. In chapter 6, I explore an example of this strategy. The performance artist Orlan has turned cosmetic surgery into an art form, whereby she claims her body as vehicle for her own identity project. I show why the attempt to treat embodied difference as something that can be altered in accordance with the individual's desires may be a powerful statement about the flexibility of postmodern identities, but of limited usefulness as critical feminist response to cosmetic surgery.

While cosmetic surgery has been associated almost exclusively with women in the past, in the wake of the enormous explosion of cosmetic surgery interventions, men appear to be altering their appearance in increasing numbers as well. Both the media and the medical profession have seized upon this phenomenon as evidence for the growing equality between the sexes, arguing that it is just a matter of time before men are having just as much cosmetic surgery as women. In chapter 7, I take issue with the notion of the "new" sexual equality in the politics of appearance. I argue for a contextual understanding of cosmetic surgery that takes the concrete particulars of individual's embodied experiences as well as historically situated, cultural discourses of difference into account.

The book closes with one of the most dramatic and unsettling applications of cosmetic surgery to eliminate embodied difference—facial surgery on Down's syndrome children to make them look "normal." It will serve as a warning to the reader that the critical inquiry into the culture of cosmetic surgery has only just begun.

NOTES

I would like to thank Anna Aalten, Willem de Haan, and Henri Wijsbek for their encouragement and helpful comments.

1. See, for example, "Our Quest to be Perfect" *Newsweek*, August 9, 1999, 52–59.
2. *Volkskrant*, March 7, 2000.

3. The debate between licensed plastic surgeons and other practitioners is a long and heated one. Beginning at the turn of the century, "beauty surgery" was regarded as the province of "quacks" and "charlatans" (see chapter 1). A more recent rendition of this controversy can be found between surgeons working in private clinics and surgeons working in a hospital setting.

4. I have particularly benefited from the work of Bordo (1993), Wiegman (1995), Haraway (1997), and Lury (2000).

5. Joan Scott (1992) certainly deserves credit for this development with her seminal critique of feminist uses (and abuses) of "experience." While her work was an important corrective for treating experience as an authentic or trustworthy source of knowledge and has been taken up by many postmodern feminists as an argument against essentialism and foundationalism, it has led to an inattentiveness to how experiences get constructed in individuals' narratives, which has been detrimental to feminist scholarship.

6. After discussing the relative merits of Bordo's and my approach in my women's studies classes, I have come to the conclusion that these are precisely the questions that need to be discussed in order to develop a cultural critique of cosmetic surgery. In this sense, our positions are—as my students have never tired of pointing out—complementary rather than opposed.

7. See McNay (2000) for an excellent account of the implications of these debates for feminist gender theory.

8. Interestingly, Bordo has no criticism of Giddens's use of the term "cultural dope." In fact, she praises him for uncovering the recursive and reproductive features of society and showing that "socialization" does not occur behind people's backs but requires their active and knowledgeable participation (Bordo 1993, 303–4).

9. This paradox is elaborated in chapter 4.

10. In a discussion at the Hastings Center where we were both present, Bordo acknowledged, for example, that "of course, it's a good thing that you talked to those women," but then went on to emphasize the necessity of focusing on structures rather than the words of individual women.

11. Ricoeur draws on Karl Jaspers's notion of "loving conflict" to describe the dangers of consensus ("if we miss consensus, we think we have failed"), the impossibility of a common or identical history, and the importance of assuming and living conflicts as a kind of practical wisdom (Ricoeur 1999, 12).

1

Cosmetic Surgery in a Different Voice: The Case of Madame Noël

The primary requisite for a good surgeon is to be a man—a man of courage.

—Edmund Andrews, "The Surgeon"

Surgery involves bodies—those of surgeons as well as of patients. . . . What does it mean when the body of the surgeon—the intrusive gazer, the violator, the recipient of sensory assaults—is that of a woman?

—Joan Cassell, *The Surgeon in the Woman's Body*

When I began my research on cosmetic surgery, I assumed that it was a fairly recent phenomenon. I vaguely remembered reading about breast augmentations in the early sixties when Carol Doda, a topless dancer in California, made the headlines by having silicone injected directly into her breasts. The enormous expansion of cosmetic surgery procedures in the years that followed seemed to be a typical by-product of Western culture in late modernity—a culture where medical technology has made the surgical alteration of the body a readily available and socially acceptable "choice" and where the belief in the makeability of the body reigns supreme. As my research progressed, however, I discovered that cosmetic surgery was not nearly as recent as I had initially imagined. In fact, it was highly popular at the turn of the century, and, to my surprise, one of the pioneers was a woman—a French surgeon, known to her colleagues as Madame Noël. She practiced during the period that cosmetic surgery was becoming a respectable branch of medicine and wrote one of the first medical handbooks about cosmetic surgery in 1926, thereby laying the groundwork for the profession as we know it today (Rogers 1971). Madame Noël was not only a cosmetic surgeon, however. She was also a feminist: a suffragette, an advocate of women's right to work, and one of the founders of Soroptimism, an international women's organization.

I was intrigued. Who was this woman and how did she manage to reconcile the seemingly irreconcilable: being a feminist and being a cosmetic surgeon? After all, cosmetic surgery, like all forms of surgery, is today a male-dominated medical specialty.[1] Female cosmetic surgeons are few and far between. Surgery is inhospitable to women, in part, because its long training period and demanding work schedules make it difficult to combine career and family. However, the surgical ethos appears to be notoriously masculine as well. The anthropologist Joan Cassell (1991) has studied surgeons at work and concludes that, as a group, they tend to be arrogant, adventurous, ruthless, and competitive. In short, surgeons possess characteristics that in Western culture tend to be associated with men and masculinity.[2] As Cassell puts it, to be a surgeon, one has to be—literally and figuratively—"ballsy" (35). While practitioners in "softer" specialties like internal medicine or general practice are like statesmen waiting to see how the illness progresses and trying with pills and potions to cooperate with the body, the surgeon behaves like a warrior, armed to the teeth. He acts (or cuts) first and thinks later. The world of surgery is a dog-eat-dog world, and surgeons tend to be highly competitive with one another. Surgeons are the consummate machos of the medical world, according to Cassell. They are prepared to operate for seven hours without a break, look down on people who complain or look tired, and generally like to "live on the edge" (Cassell 1991, 42–43). Surgeons belong to the masculine world of fast cars and sports, and many hold intensely polarized views of women as either the "nice" women they marry or the "bad" women they "play around with" (Cassell 1991, 41).

Given the "masculine" underpinnings of cosmetic surgery as a medical specialty as well as the role it plays in the inferiorization of women through their bodies, a feminist cosmetic surgeon would seem to be a contradiction in terms. It is hard to imagine how a feminist could become a cosmetic surgeon or, by the same token, how cosmetic surgery could be practiced in a way that is not, by definition, disempowering or demeaning to women.

In this chapter, I will explore this unlikely combination, using Madame Noël as an example of what can happen when a feminist woman engages in the most masculine profession of all—cosmetic surgery. Although she represents only one case, her case provides a glimpse of a surgical ethos and practice that differ considerably from what Cassell found among modern-day surgeons. After taking a brief look at Noël's life and the context in which she practiced cosmetic surgery, I examine the handbook she wrote in 1926, *La Chirurgie esthétique, son rôle social*, in which she describes her views about her profession, her techniques and procedures, and the results of her operations. In conclusion, I tackle the question of whether Noël's approach might be regarded as a "feminine" or even feminist way of doing surgery—an instance of surgery in "a different voice"[3] and what this might mean for a feminist critique of cosmetic surgery as, almost by definition, "bad news" for women.

MADAME NOËL

The life and work of Suzanne Noël have been recounted by Paule Regnault (1971), who studied surgery with her from 1942 to 1950,[4] and Jeannine Jacquemin (1988), who was commissioned by Soroptimism International to write a biography of Noël as one of the Soroptimism "founding mothers." Both provide glowing accounts of Noël as a courageous and unusual woman, a highly skilled and original surgeon, and a famous and respected apostle of the international women's movement.

Suzanne Blanche Marguerite Gros was born in 1878 in Laon, France, of well-to-do parents. As the only surviving daughter of four children, she was doted on by her parents and received the usual education reserved for middle-class girls: classics, embroidery, and painting. At nineteen, she made a "good marriage" to a doctor nine years older than she, Henri Pertat. In 1905, she embarked on her medical studies, studies that she probably could not have undertaken without the consent and active support of her husband (Jacquemin 1988, 13). (Noël later claimed that she became a doctor in order to work with her husband in his dermatology practice.) She excelled in her studies and, following an illness and the birth of her daughter, passed the highly competitive *Internat des Hôpitaux de Paris* in 1912 as the fourth of sixty-seven students. This was an exceptional performance for a woman—one that, as her official biographer notes, "could only have been achieved by extremely hard work and a brilliant intelligence" (Jacquemin 1988, 16). In 1919, her husband died, and she married a fellow student in dermatology, André Noël, who had just returned from the front in World War I. He quickly finished his *Internat* (graduating at the bottom of his class) and handed in a thesis that was probably based on work that his wife had been doing on the *douche filiforme* (an installation for bathing patients with skin problems). Their marriage was short lived. Following the death of Suzanne's daughter, André became severely depressed, and in 1924, he threw himself into the Seine in front of his wife. Devastated, Suzanne Noël turned to her work for solace, and it was to remain her passion until her death in 1954.

Noël first became interested in cosmetic surgery in 1912 when she noticed that the famous actress Sarah Bernhardt returned from her American tour miraculously rejuvenated. (Bernhardt was, at that time, well over sixty.)

Curious, Noël began experimenting by pinching the skin of her own face in different places to see if she could get the same effect. Surprised at what she was able to accomplish, she began to experiment more seriously, operating on anesthetized rabbits whose skin is similar in "delicacy and elasticity to human skin" (Noël 1932, 7).

The advent of World War I allowed Noël to gain expertise in treating wounded soldiers for facial injuries, and in 1916 she undertook further surgical training for operating on disfiguring scars as well as her old "hobby," the rejuvenation of wrinkled faces. Noël situates the beginning of her devotion to cosmetic surgery in one of her first face-lift operations on a woman who "due to her age was not able to earn her own living"—an operation that was apparently so successful that the patient was immediately able to find a job. Noël claims to have been so impressed by this fortuitous result that she decided to make cosmetic surgery her vocation and, from that point on, did not look back (Noël 1932, 9).

Noël's medical career stretched from 1916 to 1950 and can be separated into two distinct periods. When she started practicing, plastic surgery was not an established specialty, and hospitals did not admit surgeons who did exclusively plastic surgery. Noël set up her own clinic at home, becoming one of the first cosmetic surgeons in France. Her operations were limited to minor surgery, most notably face-lifts and eyelid corrections. She apparently quickly became well known, drawing many "world-renowned persons of the fashion world and of the European aristocracy" (Regnault 1971, 134).

With the onset of World War II, she gave up her private clinic and performed operations in the Clinique des Bleuets in Paris where she could do major surgery. According to her student Regnault, Noël was a versatile surgeon who performed many different and often quite bold interventions—reshaping the breasts, slimming the abdomen and arms, excising fat from the legs, and/or eliminating wrinkles in the hand by injecting a sclerosing solution into the blood vessels. Although she is credited with initiating the Biesenburger method of mammoplasty in France, it is her technique of face-lifting, in particular the "petite opération" or "mini-lift," for which she continues to be known today (see, for example, Stephenson 1970; Rogers 1971; González-Ulloa 1985).

At a time when women were struggling to gain a foothold in the medical profession, Noël appears to have won considerable recognition for her work. She was awarded the Legion of Honor in 1928 for being a "doctor of unusual skill" whose lectures and methods were a credit to her country (Jacquemin 1988, 33). In addition to writing a widely read book about cosmetic surgery that was translated into German in 1932 (*Die Äesthetische Chirurgie und ihre soziale Bedeutung*), physicians from all over the world visited Paris to observe her work. She traveled extensively in the United States, Germany, and Austria, giving lectures and demonstrating her surgical techniques. In 1930, two documentary films showing Noël operating were made in the Charité in Berlin and later written up in *Medizinische Welt*. She was the first woman in France to become the president of a medical society—that of aesthetic morphobiology. Her name is included in most historical accounts of modern cosmetic surgery where she is referred to as "the world's first famous female cosmetic plastic surgeon" (Rogers 1971).

Noël's career as a feminist ran parallel to her professional career as cosmetic surgeon. She was an ardent believer in women's right to vote and participated in speeches and parades, wearing a ribbon on her hat with the words *Je veux voter*. In an attempt to embarrass the government so that they would give women the right to vote, she organized a strike on the payment of taxes, convincing women that they should not be paying taxes over the use of which they had no control (Jacquemin 1988, 23). She studied medicine at a time when European women still had considerable difficulty training and qualifying as doctors and was firmly committed to a woman's right to a place in the professional and business world. In 1923, she became acquainted with Soroptimism, when a representative of the rapidly growing movement in the United States visited Paris to recruit new members. Soroptimism[5] was a women's organization connected to the Rotary Clubs for men that promoted the support of professional women as well as the ideals of service and internationalism. Enthralled by the Soroptimist principles, Noël set about organizing the first chapter in Europe, which was founded in Paris in 1924. During the next thirty years, she played a crucial role in expanding the organization throughout the world. She lectured extensively, traveling as far away as China and India, using her renown as a surgeon to establish new clubs. Noël is most well known for the role she played in initiating Soroptimist organizations in Europe (she single-handedly founded chapters in eleven European capitals). She became the first president of the European Federation in 1930, and in 1943 a Noël Fund was established to sustain the expansion of international Soroptimism (Jacquemin 1988, 46). Even after she was nearly blind and well into her seventies, she continued to attend international meetings up until her death at the age of seventy-six.

In summary, the picture that emerges of Suzanne Noël based on accounts of her students and sister Soroptimists is nothing short of heroic. At first glance, it would seem that she managed to do the impossible—namely, to combine the practice of cosmetic surgery with an active commitment to feminism. But what did this combination mean for how Noël actually practiced cosmetic surgery? Before taking a closer look at her approach to cosmetic surgery, let us take a brief look at the context in which she practiced this new kind of medicine.

SURGICAL PIONEERS

Suzanne Noël belongs to a group of the early pioneers of what is now known as modern cosmetic surgery.[6] Cosmetic surgery—that is, surgery undertaken solely for reasons of appearance—emerged at the end of the nineteenth century in the United States and Europe (Germany, England, France). Plastic surgery, which includes both cosmetic or aesthetic surgery and reconstructive surgery—is much older. The first rhinoplasty (nose reconstruction) was reported in India as early as a.d. 1000. In India a thief's nose might be cut off as a form of punishment or, in the case of an adulterous Hindu wife, bitten off by the wronged husband. Gaspare Tagliacozzi, often credited as the "father of plastic surgery," wrote the first book about plastic surgery in 1597, in which he gave an illustrated account of his successful reconstruction of a young nobleman's nose that had been sliced off during a duel. Plastic surgery didn't become popular until the nineteenth century when the discovery of antisepsis and anesthesia made operations feasible, and even then, most surgeons were more interested in "cavity surgery" than in repairing the body surface (McDowell 1978). It wasn't until the beginning of the twentieth century that cosmetic surgery was performed on a large scale. Two separate but related developments account for its emergence at this particular moment in history (Haiken 1997).

The first development—often ignored in official histories of plastic surgery—was the mass beauty culture that flourished at the turn of the century. Cultural prohibitions against older women attempting to look young and beautiful were dropped, and a democratic ideology of self-improvement emerged that advocated making the tools for achieving beauty available to all women, regardless of their socioeconomic circumstances (Banner 1983). In addition to beauty parlors and hairdressers, which sprang up all over the United States, cosmetic "salons" were established where people could have their faces "lifted" and their noses corrected. Advertisements appeared in daily newspapers from surgeons expounding the wonders of cosmetic surgery.

Many of the early cosmetic surgeons operated on the fringes of the medical establishment. Cosmetic surgery was associated with "quackery"—untrained charlatans or "irregular doctors" with an eye to earning a fast buck by operating on vain and silly women who were preoccupied with their appearance. Although these surgeons were not taken seriously by the established medical professionals, they developed many of the techniques that were employed and continue to be employed by cosmetic surgeons today. Rogers (1971) argues that many of these early pioneers, in fact, showed great inventiveness and foresight but were mistakenly "brushed aside or ignored" by their surgical contemporaries.

The second development leading to the emergence of cosmetic surgery was World War I and with it large numbers of soldiers with facial damage, burns, and lost limbs who required reconstructive surgery. This gave surgeons the chance to practice their surgical techniques and gain experience in performing operations. The negative associations of bodily deformity with syphilis or divine retribution for sins committed were dispelled by the noble and deserving soldier, disfigured in the defense of his country. Plastic and reconstructive surgery became acceptable, or, as Raymond Passot, a contemporary of Noël, put it, the war gained it the "keys of the city" (Rogers 1985, 13).

Cosmetic surgery remained controversial for many early plastic surgeons — a controversy that continues to play a role in contemporary discussions about surgery for reconstructive purposes (disfigurements through birth or accident) and surgery for aesthetic reasons. However, by 1921, plastic surgeons — anxious to find a market for their newly won skills, decided to include cosmetic surgery as a subspecialty of plastic surgery. The first professional association for cosmetic surgery was established in Chicago, laying the foundation for what was later to become one of the largest specialties in American medicine (Haiken 1997).

Suzanne Noël, like many early plastic surgeons, gained experience in operating on wounded soldiers during the First World War. After the war, however, she directed her attention to a new group of patients and began operating mostly on women who wanted to improve their appearance. Like her contemporaries, she brought the fields of reconstructive and cosmetic surgery together. Like most pioneers, she was interested in gaining recognition for a new and controversial medical practice as well as perfecting its procedures and techniques. To this end, she wrote *La Chirurgie esthétique, son rôle social*, which appeared in 1926 as the fourth handbook devoted entirely to cosmetic surgery.[7] Her book not only served to sum up and document several decades of work in the newly emerging field of cosmetic surgery, but became the standard text on cosmetic surgery for many years afterward. According to Rogers (1971), Noël's book marked the end of the "pioneering period" of cosmetic surgery; since then surgeons have only been concerned with "technical variations and improvements in the operations of their predecessors" (266).

THE TEXT

Medical textbooks in the field of cosmetic surgery tend to adopt the same general format. They begin with an attempt to justify the importance of cosmetic surgery as a medical specialty. This somewhat defensive stance is due to the controversial features of cosmetic surgery — features that place the author in the position of having to explain the usefulness or desirability of surgery on an otherwise healthy patient for beauty reasons. This is followed by attention to patients' motives for having cosmetic surgery. Some attempt is made to advise the surgeon on which patients are suitable candidates for surgery and when caution is indicated. And, finally, the would-be surgeon is provided with necessary information about operation techniques as well as the kinds of results that can be expected. To this end, visual materials are provided: anatomical drawings, operation photographs, and before-and-after sequences that enable the reader to assess the results of surgery.

Noël's book (1926/1932) also has a typical textbook format and, therefore, resembles many later books on cosmetic surgery. It is divided into two parts. In the first part (roughly one-third of the book), she sets out why cosmetic surgery is important and provides several vignettes of patients who were helped by aesthetic surgery. The rest of the book (roughly two-thirds) is devoted to how she does the operations, including a description of the instruments used, various techniques for making incisions, how to do sutures and apply bandages, and the outcomes. She closes with a word on possible negative side effects and further applications of aesthetic surgery. The book is relatively short, only seventy-one pages. Its most distinctive feature is the wealth of photographs and illustrations, all of which were made by the author herself. She was one of the first cosmetic surgeons to provide photographs of the entire operation instead of the ubiquitous drawings of classical Grecian female heads, which her contemporaries seemed to prefer, where dotted lines and arrows denoted the correct location for the incision, or the more recent predilection in surgical texts for photographs of isolated body parts. Noël's book also contains a large collection of before-and-after photographs of her successful as well as her less successful operations, thereby enabling the reader to assess the results of her procedures.

I shall now take a closer look at the text, focusing on why Noël thought cosmetic surgery was important (how she justified it), how she thought it should (or should not) be done, and what constituted in her view a successful operation. By comparing her to other surgeons of her day, I will show what makes her approach to cosmetic surgery distinctive. I will then turn to the question of whether she might be viewed as a "different voice" in the history of cosmetic surgery.

JUSTIFYING COSMETIC SURGERY: "THE BITTER NEED" (NOËL 1932, 10)[8]

Noël, like her contemporaries, was a fervent believer in cosmetic surgery, describing it as a "boon to mankind" (9). While she acknowledged that, as a new profession, aesthetic surgery often met with "ridicule" or a "shrug" (10), she did not dwell on such skepticism. Unlike her contemporaries, she did not defend her specialty against the disbelieving medical establishment. Instead she announced her unshakable conviction that such attitudes would disappear as soon as surgeons understood the "bitter need" behind patients' wishes to have their appearance altered surgically (10).

The "bitter need" to which she refers is an economic one. Her patients—most of whom are women—come to her because they are afraid of losing their jobs as their faces begin to show the first signs of age. She proceeds to provide a series of dramatic "cases" that will establish her defense of cosmetic surgery: the aging opera star who is no longer asked to sing ("in spite of her fame and beautiful voice . . . she wasn't even allowed to sing without pay in hospitals for veterans," [11]), the widow who can't support her young son ("abandoned by her husband and financially ruined, she was forced to seek employment," [12]), and the seamstress in the sweatshop who wants to improve her situation by becoming a supervisor (but "like other Parisian workers, long years of hard work, insufficient sleep, and poor nutrition had taken their toll," [14]). Noël justifies her profession with sympathetic accounts of why her patients want surgery and how it makes a difference in their life circumstances.

Let us take a closer look at one of these cases—her description of a "distinguished-looking, sixty-year old woman whose former beauty is clearly visible in her countenance . . . in spite of creases and wrinkles" (10):

She comes asking me for help. The war and her old appearance have caused her to lose her job as manager of a small firm in luxury goods. Her excellent references and experience and her acknowledged good taste couldn't help her: wherever she applied for a job, she received the same answer: "We'll let you know," and that was as far as she ever got. She was in the deepest distress; I agreed to undertake the rejuvenation of her appearance.

Even after the first operation, she gathered fresh courage. I discovered just how desperately she needed my immediate help on the day I removed her stitches. She fainted and had to admit that she hadn't eaten anything for 48 hours. A meal was set before her and I encouraged her with all my powers. The next day she found some work—and it was in one of the firms where she had been so roughly treated before.

I have operated on this patient three times more in the course of a two month period.

Since then, she is able to earn her living with the same ease as for the past 15 years and she was so busy in the last three years that she didn't have time to undergo the fourth operation which I considered necessary.

I see her frequently; she has gained a remarkably youthful demeanor, together with a feeling of security that she will be able to take on what life brings. This is certainly the best payment a surgeon can receive. (10–11)

While Noël's contemporaries were wont to defend cosmetic surgery by referring to the value of beauty in abstract terms or citing the psychological distress of their patients, Noël justifies operations for social or material reasons. As the title of her book suggests, she views cosmetic surgery as a social necessity, particularly for women. She sees her vocation as a way to help women support themselves or maintain their professional positions. As a feminist, Noël was herself a staunch advocate of women's right to work and had personal experience in the obstacles facing working women in her day (she was forced to practice surgery in her home as women surgeons were not admitted to hospitals).

In her book, Noël provides tongue-in-cheek observations about her patients' husbands who are reluctant to let their wives have surgery, remarking that French men exhibit the "most strenuous resistance" to cosmetic surgery and that "the wish of their wives to preserve their beauty and youthful appearance unsettles them to a high degree." Remembering her own activities as a suffragette, Noël concludes:

> It is the same as with our right to vote. Nowhere did women meet with such headstrong resistance, nowhere was it made so difficult for them to openly admit their wish to remain young. (19–20)

She suggests that this accounts for why many women may prefer to keep their surgery a secret from their husbands. Others may engage in what Noël with unmistakable irony refers to as a "little subterfuge of war." By encouraging their husbands to have surgery to rejuvenate *their* appearance, these astute women pave the way for their own face-lifts—the strategy of "what's good for the gander is also good for the goose" (20).

In short, Noël justifies cosmetic surgery in terms of material necessity and women's right to a youthful appearance. She employs a feminist discourse that situates women's right to change an "ugly face" or "humiliating body" to their right to vote and demand political rights: a matter of being able to "choose one's own destiny" (quoted in Haywood 1985, 30). She refers to power hierarchies in gender relations in tongue-in-cheek accounts of men's resistance to change and how women might employ their feminine wiles in order to get what they want in the battle between the sexes.

TECHNIQUES AND PROCEDURES: "IT MAY BE MY WOMANLY CHARACTER WHICH LED ME TO CHOOSE THIS PARTICULAR METHOD." (57)

Noël wrote her book at a time when many of the techniques and procedures of cosmetic surgery had not yet been recorded, and many were still in an experimental stage. Like her contemporaries, she would have been concerned about staking out a claim in a new field. However, the manner in which she set out her techniques and procedures stands in marked contrast to the writings of her contemporaries.

While they used abstract or technical language in their texts and tended to position themselves as distanced observers, ready to open the body and reveal its secrets,[9] Noël's text is completely devoid of technical jargon. She writes in a refreshingly down-to-earth style, providing frequent anecdotes and humorous observations. For example, she employs the domestic metaphor of sewing to describe her technique for removing a "bag under the eyes":

> I use . . . a straight or half-curved needle and an ordinary thimble which has been sterilized like the rest of the instruments. It may be my womanly nature which led me to choose this particular method, but I believe that the opening through which a needle is thrust is less likely to be pulled out of shape if the needle receives steady support [from the thimble].
> And I have always produced perfect seams. (57)

She demystifies surgery as a craft rather than a magical power—something to be learned through practice and attention to details. Her description is accessible; she seems to be writing for colleagues with an eye toward helping them perform operations in such a way that the best possible result will be achieved rather than cornering a part of the surgical market for herself.

It was not uncommon for the pioneers of modern cosmetic surgery to give detailed accounts about which instruments to use, where to place clamps, and what kind of material should be used for suturing, or how to bandage the wound.

However, while most of these early surgeons focused on the incision—the numbing of the skin, the actual cutting, and the closing of the wound—Noël pays attention to the operation as a whole (Stephenson 1985). Beginning with the preparations for an operation, she describes experimenting with different possibilities with the patient, pulling back the skin and adjusting the direction according to the patient's wishes. She mobilizes the patient's skills in preparing the operation, asking her to experiment in front of her own mirror at home in order to see which kind of pull yields the best results.

> My experience is that the patient is always the one to find the best place [to make the incisions]. This is a small trick which I can heartily recommend to anyone doing cosmetic surgery. (24)

Once Noël had determined the best place to make the incision, she made crescent-shaped appliqué-patterns that were placed at different locations along the hairline. She developed a special measuring band called a "craniometer," which she placed at the center of the patient's forehead and used as a guide for ensuring that one side of the patient's face would be aligned with the other.

Her attention to the details of the procedure is apparent throughout her description of the operation. For example, she provides a list of the instruments to be used in the operations, including the number of each, the best kinds of needles and suturing material, and which kinds of bandages are most effective. It is almost like reading a recipe whereby the cook is given all the necessary information in order to prepare a particular dish. She reminds surgeons not to forget to check whether the patient's face is numb after administering the local anesthesia or to be sure to cover the patient with a blanket so that she won't get cold during the operation (24).

Noël took pictures of the entire procedure, beginning with the preparations (measuring the patient's skull, applying the patterns) and ending with the patient perched happily on the bed after the operation, fixing her hair or drinking a cup of coffee. In this way, the reader is given a blow-by-blow account of the operation rather than a diagram of where to place the incision. The patient is present in the photographs as is Noël herself—sometimes shown in full view, operating on the patient, or just as a hand, gently resting by the patient's head following the surgery.

Noël's concern for her patient's well-being extends beyond the actual surgery. She anticipates how the patient will have to return home after surgery and confront her family and colleagues, many of whom do not know that she has had an operation. Noël imaginatively places herself in her patient's shoes when she makes incisions behind the hairline or dyes the bandage to match the patient's hair or advises her patient to change her hairstyle or buy a new hat so that she doesn't have to explain why she looks so much better. Her goal is that her patient can "return home and immediately go about her daily activities" without having to explain her actions to curious family members or friends (37).

For most surgeons working in the first half of this century, the patient was an absent presence. Their attention was focused on the body part upon which the operation was performed. If patients appear at all in early textbooks on cosmetic surgery, it was to warn the would-be surgeon about the dangers of "feminine persuasion." For example, Eugen Holländer (1932) writes retrospectively of being a "victim" to a Polish aristocrat who insisted that he perform a face-lift on her in 1901 at a time when the operation was totally unknown (quoted in Rogers 1971, 274). Surgeons like Charles Conrad Miller elaborated the potential difficulties in managing operations with women whom he referred to as "high-strung, modern types who suffer enough from nerves already" and advised maintaining a calm and unhurried demeanor and avoiding subjecting the patient to the sight of blood (Miller 1925, quoted in Stephenson 1985, 32). In contrast, Noël treats the operation as a collaborative endeavor. The patient is present in her text as an active and knowledgeable participant in the surgery. From the initial consultation to the follow-up, she draws the patient into the procedure, making use of her ideas about how the operation should be done. She acknowledges that patients may be often "more alert" to the first signs of aging and, therefore, are in a better position than Noël to decide whether an operation is necessary (41). She never belittles nervous patients but maintains that all her patients "behave in a calm and sensible way during surgery" (10). If a patient fails to return for an additional operation, Noël notes humorously that she was probably just too busy with her job to be bothered.

In short, Noël portrays the techniques and procedures as an ordinary skill not unlike sewing. She values experience, patience, care for details, and dexterity rather than scientific knowledge and the daring incision. She is collegial toward her fellow surgeons, seemingly more intent on sharing her knowledge than taking credit for innovations. But, most important, she takes a respectful and collaborative stance toward her patients, never losing sight of the context in which they decide to have their operations as well as live with the outcome.

RISKS AND RESULTS: "THIS BRANCH OF SURGERY IS FULL OF AMBUSHES . . . CARE IS IN ORDER IF TRAGIC ACCIDENTS ARE TO BE AVOIDED." (70)

During the first half of the century, there was considerable controversy even then about the best technique for a face-lift.[10] Noël was a staunch opponent of the heroic measures favored by many of her contemporaries like Sir Harold Gillies, Robert Ivy, Otto Bames, and Erich Lexer. She advocated what she called a "petite opération" for face-lifting (also sometimes called the "timid intervention"). This involved making small elliptical excisions around the hairline where they would be invisible and suturing the skin without excising the underlying tissue. She removed just enough skin to create the necessary tension to bring about improvement. This was in contrast to her contemporaries who experimented with bolder incisions stretching from the patient's temple to behind the earlobe or advocated undermining large areas of subcutaneous tissue in the interests of a more durable result. For example, the American surgeon Otto Bames was openly disparaging of what he called the "timorousness" of "would-be surgeons" who were afraid

to adopt radical procedures (most notably, his own) in the interests of achieving "permanent results" (Bames 1927, 86, quoted in González-Ulloa 1985,
46). While Noël was not alone in her skepticism of "la grande opération,"
she was unusual in her concern for preventing scars and her cautious approach toward experimentation. Her interventions were invariably designed
with an eye to preventing scars. She preferred to do a series of smaller interventions over a period of years, sometimes doing one side of the face first
and waiting to see how it turned out before doing the other side. She believed
that it was better to leave no traces and avoid risks of blood clots or paraly-
sis of facial muscles (a potential side effect of undermining) even if it meant
having to do further surgery. She did not see the necessity of accomplishing
everything in a single operation.

Noël's contemporaries emphasized the spectacular improvements that
could be achieved with cosmetic surgery and were prepared to take serious
risks in the interest of refining their techniques. They rarely mentioned unsuccessful or failed operations.[11] Noël provides photographs of her own less-
than-satisfactory results. She devotes an entire chapter in her book to scars,
showing what could happen when incisions are inappropriately made (incisions that are not in the right place, unsightly scars due to the development of
keloid tissue, or scars where the ear lobe is pulled out of shape). For Noël,
scars were not an unavoidable accoutrement to surgery, nor did she blame the
patient for being too picky. She readily admitted that her work was experimental and that she often began an operation without quite knowing what she
was getting into. However, she seems less cavalier than many of her contemporaries about the dangers of her interventions. For example, in describing
one of her first operations, she notes that her patient, a man, "stoically refused
to be anaesthetized" and that she made mistakes that not only complicated the
procedure, but caused the operation to last longer than planned and the wound
to heal more slowly. Fortunately, the results were excellent and, in hindsight,
she notes that this was the operation during which she "learned more than all
the others that followed" (8).

Some of her operations did fail, of course. This is not surprising, given that
Noël performed operations at a time when surgeons did not have access to
some of the technology available today and when precautions to avoid infec-
tion were less stringent. For example, Noël's book contains numerous photos
of her operating on her patients without gloves, and one of her students re-
members that Noël left her watch on her wrist during surgery and told her
laughingly afterward not to worry because "this watch is very good" (Regnault 1971, 137).

Noël was apparently devastated by her more serious failures, however. For
example, a "leg defatting" turned out so badly that she worried about it for a

long time afterward, tending to justify herself and speak in a "very sharp tone that even her friends recognized" (Jacquemin 1988, 33).

On the whole, Noël's results were surprisingly good. According to Regnault (1971),

> the delicate way in which she handled the tissues (avoiding forceps, pressure, and tension) was certainly a great factor in her good results. If she were alive today, her surgical technique would certainly include the latest advances, but her basic philosophy about the place of esthetic surgery would undoubtedly be the same as it always was. (13)

It was Noël's attention to the results and her desire to avoid side effects that enabled her to achieve outcomes that, judging by the photographs of her patients, were at least as good as many of the face-lifts performed today. Although Noël might have modified her "timid" procedure had she lived longer, it seems unlikely that she would have ever adopted the heroic stance toward cosmetic surgery favored by her male colleagues. As she herself put it, there would probably always be women who would forgo a more dramatic improvement if it meant that their working or living situations would not be disrupted. For these patients, two or three operations over a period of several years would be preferable to the single, more radical intervention. For Noël, patients were individuals with different needs and desires. Even if more radical interventions were advisable from a surgical point of view, it should still be left to the individual woman to decide. A woman's special circumstances might advise against radical surgery, causing her to choose surgery that doesn't "show" and that can easily be integrated into her current life situation. In her view, the patient, not the surgeon, is the final arbiter.

GENDER AND THE SURGICAL ETHOS

The surgical ethos described at the beginning of this article is not limited to modern-day surgeons, but is echoed in the writings of the early pioneers as well. González-Ulloa (1985) prefaces his history of cosmetic surgery by calling it:

> a story of discovery. It describes how *men* [my italics] explored and charted the realm of possibilities, bringing into existence new activities which today—in our present age—constitute an integrated geographical guide to the possible. (González-Ulloa 1985, i)

Early cosmetic surgeons like Charles Conrad Miller, Jacques Joseph, or Otto Bames maintained and helped construct the image of the cosmetic surgeon as a rugged, male explorer, embarking on exciting adventures in unknown territory. These men were lonely heroes who were highly competitive and did not hesitate to take credit for one another's discoveries (Rogers 1971). The first books on cosmetic surgery were full of daring experiments of medical men who were more interested in novel solutions than careful trial and error. They tended to treat their patients as mere objects for their scientific endeavors, and some were quick to ridicule their patients as vain society women engaged in the trivial pursuit of beauty. A case in point was Charles Conrad Miller, the first surgeon to write a textbook about cosmetic surgery, who was well known for his "megalomania" and "messianic egotism" and who quite literally believed that he could do no wrong (Rogers 1971, 267). Miller experimented with various questionable materials for facial implants, including braided silk, sponge rubber, pieces of ivory or gutta-percha that he ground up in an ordinary spinach grinder. He injected paraffin into his patient's faces and daringly advocated cutting facial nerves and muscles as a preventative measure against "expression lines" to which he believed women were particularly prone (Miller 1923, quoted in Rogers 1971, 269; Haiken 1997, 25) . He also ran afoul of the law for illegal ownership of quack drug stores in Chicago and selling narcotics without prescriptions. Nevertheless, medical historians still refer to Miller as "something of a surgical visionary years ahead of his more academic colleagues" (Rogers 1971, 266) or give him credit for acknowledging the social forces that drove many women to the surgeon's office and for convincing his colleagues not to laugh off their patients' desire to improve their appearance (Haiken 1997, 25–29). A surgeon's faults seem to fade in the light of his contribution to the development of a profession—a profession that apparently demands a certain amount of arrogance and audacity.

With her characteristic views on the profession and practice of cosmetic surgery, Madame Noël represents a radical departure from both her contemporaries and her successors. She stands in sharp contrast to the archetypal surgeon described by Cassell (1991)—that invincible hero imbued with all the "right stuff" required to get the job done. Noël was not only a woman working in a man's world, but she displayed an ethos that did not fit the values and behavior that have historically been regarded as the sine qua non of surgery.

Like the other pioneers of cosmetic surgery, Noël was interested in promoting and developing her field. Like them, she was also involved in experimenting with new techniques and procedures. However, she was also cautious, going to great lengths to avoid taking unnecessary risks. She was enthusiastic about her profession, but never arrogant, and invariably prepared to admit that she made mistakes. She situated herself as a craftswoman rather than a magician with mysterious powers to transform the human body. Her goal was to teach and communicate rather than to stake out her territory and set herself apart from other surgeons. She did not describe her operations as a public spectacle where the surgeon has to cut first and think later. Instead she depicted surgery as a rather mundane event, not unlike cooking a meal or sewing a seam, requiring patience, experience, and a "good eye." Noël was less obsessed with the incision as the surgeon's moment of glory than with the operation as a whole—a process that began before the patient arrived in her office for the first time and ended months or even years after the first intervention. For her, the immediate result of the operation was less important than the long-term consequences for the patient who also might need time to reconsider her options or decide that she was too busy for further surgery.

Noël does not appear as a lonely discoverer, exploring the secrets of the human body. Instead she seems to be engaged in an ongoing and highly collaborative interaction with the patient—from giving the prospective candidate patterns to try out at home to the gentle hand resting on her patient's shoulder (as depicted in photographs of the operations) to her unflagging interest in the patient's successes and misfortunes during the years that followed. Noël was not only respectful of her patients' wishes, but had no qualms about conceding that a patient might know better than the surgeon what was required. And, last but not least, Noël was especially sympathetic to her women patients. She took a personal interest in their problems and understood their reasons for wanting cosmetic surgery. She situated their desire to have their faces rejuvenated or their bodies improved in the difficulties that women of her day had obtaining and holding onto paid employment. For Noël, cosmetic surgery was just as much a right for women as their right to work or even to vote.

In short, Madame Noël provides a glimpse of another kind of professionality and professional practice. If the ethos of surgery is typically "masculine," then Noël's surgical ethos could be viewed as drawing upon values that have often been associated with femininity: empathy, patience, a concern for the particularities of each case, and a modesty about her accomplishments that allowed her to share her success with her colleagues and entertain self-doubt (Keller 1983). As such, her case might be regarded as an example of cosmetic surgery in a different voice.

CAN A FEMINIST BE A COSMETIC SURGEON?

At the outset of this chapter, I raised the question of whether a feminist could possibly be a cosmetic surgeon or, more generally, whether practicing cosmetic surgery would, by definition, be antithetical to the values of feminism. Feminists are critical of cosmetic surgery, not only because it is dangerous, but also for ideological reasons. At best, it may provide temporary relief for

an individual woman's problems with her appearance. At worst, cosmetic surgery represents a capitulation to the cultural norms that victimize women in
the name of beauty. As such, cosmetic surgery is often viewed as "unalterably
opposed" to the goals of liberation and emancipation that are the bread and
butter of feminism (Haiken 1997, 275).

Madame Noël practiced at a time when cosmetic surgery was a marginal
and slightly disreputable medical specialty that was valiantly trying to gain
acceptance in the mainstream of medicine. "First-wave" feminism in France
and elsewhere was primarily concerned with issues like suffrage, access to
education, women's right to paid employment, or the protection of poor
women from prostitution or deplorable conditions in factories and sweatshops
(Boxer 1982). Beauty was not a major issue for feminists of the first wave,
with the notable and somewhat eccentric exception of Amelia Bloomer and
the clothing reformers who campaigned against the constricting corset and
unwieldy skirts dictated by high fashion in favor of loosely fitting clothing.[12]
It would be anachronistic to dismiss Noël because she did not subscribe to the
present critique of cosmetic surgery as put forth by feminists in response to
the current proliferation of technologies for body improvement and the cultural pressures on women to meet the ideals of feminine beauty. In order to
assess Noël's contribution as a cosmetic surgeon and the relevance of her
work for a feminist critique of cosmetic surgery, we need to situate both
her feminism and her medical practice in the context in which she practiced.

As feminist, Noël belonged to a women's organization that was concerned, first and foremost, with gaining access to work, particularly work in
the professions. Although Noël was sensitive to the economic pressures
affecting women of all classes (she claimed, for example, that she was prepared to operate free of charge for her less affluent patients), she did not
question the norms that made aging women seem unfit for employment or
legitimated men abandoning their wives in favor of younger women. She
poked fun at men for obstructing their wives' desire to improve themselves
but advised her patients to employ the "feminine" strategies of manipulation or deceit rather than direct confrontation. While Noël might have
adopted the stance of some of her feminist contemporaries that beauty—
particularly fashion—was trivial compared to the more pressing issues of
emancipation, it is unlikely that this would have changed her belief in
women's right to improve their appearance. She was convinced that cosmetic surgery alleviated suffering and was a useful tool for helping
women—to be sure, affluent, professional women—to achieve financial in-
dependence and social recognition.

As such, Noël's vision of cosmetic surgery might seem to have little relevance for present feminist critiques of the feminine beauty system and the

role cosmetic surgery plays in disciplining and normalizing women through their bodies. We might conclude that advocating a woman's right to a youthful face does little to dismantle the inequities of a society that treats older women as unfit for work. Noël's uncritical belief in cosmetic surgery as a solution to women's professional problems might seem to represent a feminism of compliance and accommodation rather than a feminism of rebellion and resistance.

It is my contention, however, that such conclusions would be short sighted, particularly if we situate Noël's work in the context of medicine. It is here that her views on cosmetic surgery, the techniques and procedures she developed, as well as her ideas about how operations should be performed, can be seen as a radical departure from medical practice, both in her own day and at present. Her approach to cosmetic surgery provides a dramatic antidote to the masculine ethos of surgery with its preference for the "heroic" intervention, its lack of concern for embodied realities of patients' circumstances, and, last but not least, its reticence to be critical of its own practices. In view of the current expansion of medical technologies for altering the body and the medical profession's willingness to act first and think about the consequences later, Noël's approach to cosmetic surgery is a timely reminder of the continuing importance of combining "sympathy with science" (Morantz-Sanchez 1985). She provides a vision of a different kind of medical practice—a practice that is respectful, responsible, and reflexive.

It is here that we should look for Madame Noël's feminist contribution—not in her attempts to empower individual women through face-lifts, but rather in the kind of professionality that she represented. While this may not be enough for a feminist cosmetic surgery, it is an ingredient that a feminist critique of cosmetic surgery should not ignore.

NOTES

I would like to thank Willem de Haan, Barbara Henkes, renée hoogland, and Dubravka Zarkov for their thoughtful comments on an earlier version of this chapter. I am also indebted to Ms. Bakker-Leentvaar of the Soroptimist organization in the Netherlands for her help.

1. In 1995, 23.5 percent of specialists in family medicine and 30 percent of gynecologists were women, while female surgeons remained few and far between: 8.8 percent of general surgeons, 8.7 percent of plastic surgeons, 2.5 percent of urological surgeons, and only .02 percent of thoracic surgeons (American Medical Association 1996–1997). As of 2001, the number of women plastic surgeons is estimated to be 1 in 9 (*Plastic Surgery Information Service,* Expanded Version 2001 Statistics).

2. "Masculine" is not the same as gender specific. Cassell (1991) observes that many male surgeons do not display the "right stuff" that epitomizes the ethos of surgery, while some women will. Culturally, however, the values and behavior that exemplify the ideal surgeon are perceived as masculine, just as the prototypical patient is associated with stereotypical "feminine" qualities like dependency or frailty.

3. I borrow this term from Carol Gilligan's (1982) well-known *In a Different Voice* about gender differences in morality and women's great propensity to adopt an ethic of care.

4. Regnault (1971) describes meeting the—by then—sixty-four-year-old Noël in 1942 as follows:

> She was sitting at a desk in a consulting room at the Clinique des Bleuets and wearing a black feather hat and black coat. She looked exactly as she appears in the picture reproduced here. She had a smooth and oval face without a wrinkle—having herself had multiple face lifts and blepharoplasties. . . . I was impressed by her dignity. She gave, at once, the impression of being a grand lady—although she was no more than 5 feet 4 inches high. . . . her words were simple and direct. They revealed a clear mind. . . . wisdom, calmness, and self-confidence emerged from her appearance and manner. (133–34)

5. The term Soroptimist combines *soeur* (sister/woman) with optima to mean, literally, the "best for women." See Haywood (1985) for a history of the international Soroptimist movement.

6. Among the early pioneers of cosmetic surgery are Charles Conrad Miller, Frederick Strange Kolle, Eugen Holländer, Erich Lexer, Raymond Passot, Adalbert G. Bettman, Julien Bourguet, Jacques Joseph, Harold Napier Lyons Hunt, and Suzanne Noël. See, Stephenson 1970; Rogers 1971; Regnault 1971; González-Ulloa 1985.

7. The first medical article on a cosmetic operation is thought to have been written by John Roe of Rochester, New York, in 1887. It was called "The Deformity Termed 'Pug Nose' and Its Correction by a Simple Operation." Papers appeared in the early 1900s on nose corrections, eyelid surgery and face-lifting. The first full-length medical history of cosmetic surgery was written by Charles Conrad Miller from Chicago in 1907, and a slightly expanded version appeared in 1908. Frederick Strange Kolle, a German-born American, was the second to write a medical history of cosmetic surgery in 1911, and his book was much more extensive—"a large tome consisting of 511 pages and 522 illustrations" (Rogers 1971).

8. All further references to *La Chirurgie esthétique* in this section are indicated by page number only and are taken from the German translation.

9. Take, for example, Julien Bourguet's popular treatise on the correction of "baggy eyelids" (1928), which is described at length in Stephenson (1985, 32–37). He uses language like "herniated intraorbital fat" and "mucosa of the conjunctival cul-de-sac," speaks in the first person plural ("If we examine figure 1 we realize that there are some emptinesses in certain places"), and, generally, positions himself as someone viewing the patient's body, ready to dissect it and uncover its secrets.

10. The "mini-lift" has been the subject of some controversy among cosmetic surgeons. Stephenson (1970) traces the history, showing how Noël's intervention was

replicated in the "fifteen-minute tuck," which was popular in the late sixties. The controversy continues to be waged over the best method for face-lifting. Given the fact that even extensive face-lifts usually have to be redone, it seems likely that the final word has yet to be said on the subject of the face-lift.

11. This has not changed. It wasn't until 1972 that Robert Goldwyn compiled the first collection of papers devoted to the "unfortunate result" in cosmetic surgery and attempted to explain practitioners' reluctance to deal with their mistakes.

12. Not all feminists were in favor of clothing reform, as they found new fashions like bloomers unfitting for respectable women. Moreover, arguments for more comfortable clothing were framed in terms of health rather than beauty, and, indeed, considerable attention was directed at devising fashionable reform clothing. See Newton (1974).

2

Lonely Heroes and Great White Gods: Medical Stories, Masculine Stories

Plastic surgery is one of the most "gendered" of all medical specialties. While the typical recipient of plastic surgery is likely to be a woman (more than 91 percent of all patients are women), the surgeon is almost always a man. Only about 1 in 9 plastic surgeons are women.[1] The gender gap in medical specialties like plastic surgery tends to be explained with reference to the incompatibility of long internships, irregular hours, and the demands of child rearing on women. However, the culture of a medical specialty can also be masculine, making it more appealing to men than to women. In his analysis of masculinity in various professions, David Morgan (1981, see also 1992) has noted that gender tends to be ignored when it comes to understanding men in male-dominated professions. While gender is frequently invoked in research on women's activities, men's activities tend to be described in gender-neutral terms. He illustrates this by drawing self-critically upon his own earlier research in which he collected biographies of Anglican bishops. While he originally linked the massive maleness of the episcopacy and the clergy to factors like economic and social status, he later wonders whether many of the typical traits that he discovered in these biographies were not simply instances of masculinity "in episcopal robes" (Morgan 1981, 88). Thus, he argues that we need to reflect on how professional values are conflated with and reinforce notions about masculinity and femininity.

In this chapter, I propose to explore the gendered underpinnings of the profession of cosmetic surgery.[2] It is my contention that if women's decisions to undergo cosmetic surgery can be linked to the practices and discourses of femininity—as I have argued in the past (Davis 1995), then men's decisions to perform cosmetic surgery should also bear a connection to the practices

and discourses of masculinity. As illustration, I shall examine a popular autobiography by a male plastic surgeon titled *Doctor Pygmalion* (Maltz 1954).
By analyzing the textual practices, which the author employs to construct his
life as the idealized story of plastic surgeon, the professional ideology of plastic surgery as well as the construction of masculinity in its professionalized
form can be explored.

AUTOBIOGRAPHIES AS CULTURAL TEXTS

Autobiographies are a popular genre in contemporary Western culture. They
allow readers to escape from their humdrum existence by reading about the
lives of the rich and famous. In addition to giving ordinary people a glimpse
of the desires, struggles, and accomplishments of their idols, past and present,
popular autobiographies enable readers to give meaning to their own lives.
They offer idealized models of the "good life"—models that furnish direction, sanction deviation, and provide standards against which people can measure and judge their own life course (Gergen and Gergen 1993, 194).

In recent years, social scientists have begun to draw upon popular autobiographies as a resource for understanding social life. Autobiographies provide
insight into the ideologies of a particular culture (Plummer 1983 and 1995;
Denzin 1989; Gergen and Gergen 1993; Stanley 1993; Stanley and Morgan
1993). When individuals write their autobiographies, they are not simply providing factual accounts of their lives. Rather they assemble various events,
characters, and behaviors in such a way that a certain kind of "self" is produced. In most autobiographies, the chief emphasis is on success (in some
cases, success in overcoming some adversity like illness or poverty). The narrator positions herself or himself as an expert—the wiser and more powerful
person who sets out to "edify" the reader in what it means to be an extraordinary person or to have lived a noteworthy life. Autobiographies are embedded
in the historical, cultural, and social context in which they are produced,
thereby providing valuable insight into the ideals, aspirations, but also contradictions and ambivalences of that culture.

Within feminist scholarship, autobiographies have been taken up as a significant way to recover the experiences of the powerless, most notably,
women. Attention has been focused on the different ways women and men
tell their life stories (Brodzki and Schenck 1988; Personal Narratives Group
1989; Gergen and Gergen 1993). Autobiographies have also been treated as
an object for investigating (and deconstructing) gender as textual practice
(Stanley 1993). They allow us to understand how the ideologies of masculinity and femininity are implicated in the construction of ideal selves.

Doctor Pygmalion is not a typical autobiography. While most popular autobiographies are about famous individuals (well-known historical personages, politicians, literary figures, artists, scientists, inventors, film stars, or musicians), Maxwell Maltz, although clearly successful, is not famous. At first glance, his autobiography seems to be just a straightforward "rags-to-riches" story about a poor American youth who embarks upon a career. It is a tale of a mundane hero in single-minded pursuit of one goal: to become a plastic surgeon. However, *Doctor Pygmalion* is a career story with a twist.

Doctor Pygmalion is situated in the period when plastic surgery had just begun to make its entrance as a legitimate branch of medicine. During the period between 1900 and 1925, plastic surgery became popular in the United States and Europe. It was advertised in daily newspapers and weeklies along with products like "bust creams," abdominal supporters, or chin straps designed to facilitate rejuvenation and attractiveness. "Cosmetic surgery parlors" lured thousands of women for face-lifts, eyelid corrections, and nose jobs. Many of these early operations were performed by charlatans or physicians without any training in plastic surgery. However, the line was a thin one as many trained surgeons borrowed the techniques and procedures devised by the "quacks," taking credit for them in scholarly articles (Rogers 1971). The first scientific articles and textbooks chronicling the development of cosmetic surgery appeared in the early 1920s in Europe and the United States. *Doctor Pygmalion* opens in 1925, when Maltz decides to become a plastic surgeon, and takes the author through World War II, when he has reached the pinnacle of his career.

Unlike most popular autobiographies, it contains all of the ingredients of a medical textbook on plastic surgery. Each chapter contains a combination of personal stories taken from the author's life and technical, highly detailed descriptions of surgical procedures, replete with blow-by-blow accounts of operations and even details on the kinds of surgical instruments that are employed for the various techniques. The book is full of case studies, and, indeed, most of the characters have been or are about to become the author's patients. At regular intervals, the story of his career is interrupted with historical sketches of how plastic surgery developed, illustrated with drawings of surgical instruments and procedures, which were used in the early days of plastic surgery. Numerous references and anecdotes are provided about the "founding fathers" of plastic surgery. Before-and-after photographs of a variety of procedures are available (surgery for cleft palate, receding chin, or webbed fingers; nose and ear corrections; face-lifts) with a note that, for reasons of privacy, they do not include actual patients of Maxwell Maltz. In fact, the only "personal" photograph in the book is a frontispiece portrait of Maltz, taken at the end of his career.[3]

This hybrid format enables Maltz to interweave his personal story with the story of his profession. His ambitions, values, and accomplishments become intertwined with the developments, discourses, and practices of plastic surgery. His career trajectory is reflected in the emergence and development of plastic surgery as a legitimate medical specialty. Personal accounts of his youth or relationships with family and friends are mobilized to illustrate his socialization into the world of plastic surgery, thereby reproducing its discourses of professionality. When the author presents himself as an adventurous pioneer, an idealistic man of science, or a compassionate physician, he also constructs his specialty as an exciting, revolutionary, and worthy field of medicine. In presenting his life as an exemplary plastic surgeon, Maltz simultaneously constructs an idealized image of his profession—an image that represents the ideological underpinnings of plastic surgery.

Before turning to the construction of masculinity in *Doctor Pygmalion* as well as the interconnections between masculinity and the discourses and practices of plastic surgery, let us take a brief look at the author's autobiography.

THE STORY

Maxwell Maltz ("Maxie") was born in 1899 on the "wild and woolly" Lower East Side in New York, the only son of "formidably respectable," lower-middle-class Jewish parents. After his father's early death, Maltz's mother sells her pearl choker so that her son can become a specialist. The decision to become a plastic surgeon is taken when Maltz, still an intern, delivers a baby with a harelip to a horrified young couple living in the tenements. Determined to combat what he sees as traditional views—deformities as "evidence of the displeasure of God for some grievous sin long since committed" (11)—Maltz embarks upon his career in the "very noble and compassionate form of the practice of medicine"—plastic surgery (12). As plastic surgery was still very much in its beginning stages during the early 1920s, there was plenty of room for an idealistic and ambitious young man like Maltz. He decides to pack his bags and go to Berlin for his internship.[4]

In 1923, he enters the clinic in Berlin as an intern and studies under two professors. The first was a "frosty" aristocrat, Professor von Eicken, who was known for having performed an operation on Hitler's throat. The second was Jacques Joseph, who has been called the "father of the nose correction" and whose techniques are still referred to in handbooks of cosmetic surgery. Sander Gilman devotes an entire chapter of his book *The Jew's Body* (1991) to this man (dubbed "Nosef" in fin de siècle Berlin society) who was famous for reducing "Jewish noses" to gentile proportions. Gilman describes him as an "acculturated Jew" who changed his name from Jakob to Jacques and belonged to ultraconservative fraternities where dueling was a sign of manliness. He himself bore several scars on his face as a sign that he had become integrated into German society. His scars ultimately didn't help him. Depressed at the Hitlerian threats and persecution, he committed suicide in 1934 at the age of sixty-nine by shooting himself in the mouth. Maltz makes no references to tensions that must have been present in the clinic, nor does he indicate that his own Jewishness causes any difficulties in his interactions with his teachers. On the contrary, he invariably refers to them in admiring terms, as "redoubtable men" (19) whom he wishes to emulate (by adopting their techniques or growing a mustache). Evidently, the context in which he works fades in importance against his burning ambition to become a plastic surgeon.

During his internship, Maltz meets the love of his life, a beautiful and rich American pianist, Sylvia. He travels around Europe with her as she gives concerts, earning his way by demonstrating the art of the nose job. Maltz and Sylvia plan to marry, and he returns to New York to set up his practice and buy an apartment. Just as he has made all the arrangements, he receives a note from Sylvia that she has found another man who "needed her more." Momentarily heartbroken, but undeterred, Maltz recruits his first patient and, from then on, his career as a plastic surgeon takes off.

By 1927 he already has a booming practice among the wealthy inhabitants of New York despite the Great Depression, and by 1934, he moves his practice to a penthouse and is treating actresses, celebrities, and socialites. He hires a butler and gives parties to which the Gershwins are invited. Although he briefly contemplates marriage, he remains a bachelor, unable to find a woman who can compare with the beautiful Sylvia. While Maltz clearly enjoys his success, he also writes that he suffers occasionally from pangs of conscience at the many wealthy women who demanded to have their already-beautiful noses corrected or their still-youthful faces lifted. Anxious that he has strayed from his initial idealism ("the noble and compassionate practice of medicine") by treating such trivial complaints, he assuages his moral qualms about his professional practice by offering his services to the poor for free, often recruiting them from his old neighborhood on the Lower East Side.

In the early 1940s, Maltz—like most plastic surgeons—was caught up in the war effort and spent his time lecturing on the latest techniques in reconstructive and plastic surgery in military hospitals throughout the United States.[5] After the war, he embarks upon his "most ambitious medical undertaking so far," which involves traveling to Central and South American as an ambassador of "inter-American medical good will" (221) where he operates on "indigent people" and teaches his colleagues how to perform plastic surgery. Having reached the pinnacle of his career (Maltz was fifty-five years old when he published his autobiography), he ends the book on a personal note. Upon returning from one of his trips, he discovers a young woman in his waiting room with an astonishing resemblance to his old flame, Sylvia. Lo and behold, this woman turns out to be none other than Sylvia's daughter, who has come to pay her respects now that she lives in New York. Upon closer inspection, the resemblance to her beautiful mother is marred by her sagging lower lip, a "deformity" which she has unfortunately inherited from her father. Maltz characteristically takes the initiative and offers to operate on Sylvia's daughter for free. As he magnanimously puts it when he calls the mother, "I have a purely selfish reason. . . . I want to pretend she's *my* [his italics] daughter—yours and mine. And how can I possibly do that if every time I look at her I see her real father looking back at me?" (223). The operation takes place and is successful. The young woman seems to be pleased with her new face, and Maltz feels that if "only in a small measure" she "really was mine" and that he had "won out" over his old rival after all (223). On that note, the book ends.

IDENTITY CONSTRUCTIONS

In writing his autobiography, Maxwell Maltz is not simply providing an account of the facts of his life. Indeed, the reader frequently wonders just how true to life his autobiography actually is. The events of his life are constructed in such a way that he can underline the wonders of his profession and defend it against would-be critics. Maltz is also continuously engaged in the business of self-presentation. *Doctor Pygmalion* contains various intertwining stories, which, in turn, provide different versions of the kind of person Maxwell Maltz is. For example, it is a success story about a poor Jewish boy, who like many American immigrants, pulls himself up by the bootstraps. There is the story of the adventurous physician who ventures out into unknown territory by taking up a new medical specialty. It is the story of a socially engaged physician and his struggles to avoid being corrupted by money and success and remain true to the ideals of his profession. And, last but not least, *Doctor Pygmalion* is the story of a man in search of the perfect woman. While these stories provide different constructions of self, they are unified under one primary identity: the identity of a plastic surgeon. Maltz goes to great lengths to present himself as a representative of this profession.

I shall now take a closer look at the various "selves" that are constructed in *Doctor Pygmalion*: the pioneer, the scientist, the idealist, the creator, and the aesthete and show how each works toward creating a specific professional identity—the ideal plastic surgeon.

Pioneer

Maltz presents himself as a pioneer who must contend with the misunderstanding and prejudices of the medical mainstream and the general public in order to win acceptance for a new field. He complains about "traditional" views about physical deformities as punishment from God, to be accepted with impunity, rather than a problem, which can be easily treated by "modern" surgical methods (11). Another misconception is that plastic surgeons are disreputable charlatans out to make a quick buck rather than "real" doctors. When he informs his mother that he wants to become a plastic surgeon, she is incensed, referring to his beloved vocation as being a *"beauty* [his italics] doctor, a movie-picture kind of doctor, not a real doctor, like the man who pulled out tonsils and cured scarlet fever" (12). His mother is not the only person who is skeptical of plastic surgery. Maltz must continually undermine these prejudices and reinstate the image of his field as a legitimate and commendable branch of medicine. He does this by showing that his patients do not fit the stereotypical notions of plastic surgery as frivolous "vanity work," something for "fur-clad ladies." For example, when the director of the clinic in which he works denies him a bed for his patient with the argument: "If she wants to have you make her face prettier, why doesn't she stop buying lipsticks and save her money until she can afford it?" Maltz points out that his patient is a young girl with a disfiguring burn: "She hasn't got into the lipstick habit yet. She's eight" (52). Or, he invites his colleagues who disapprove of his "new-fangled ideas" (66) to operations in which he dazzles them with his technical skill, forcing them to admit that his specialty is a worthwhile addition to medicine.

Somewhat paradoxically, Maltz underlines his status as a pioneer in plastic surgery by referring to his forebear Tagliacozzi, an Italian nobleman who is regarded as the "father of plastic surgery."[6] This early plastic surgeon started doing nose reconstructions as early as 1597 on individuals who had lost their noses as a result of disease (leprosy, syphilis) or punishment or, in one case, an accident while dueling. Although his methods inspired plastic surgeons up into the twentieth century, he was considered a heretic in his time and, in fact, was ultimately killed during the Inquisition. The implication is that Maltz, like Tagliacozzi, is more enlightened than his more pedestrian colleagues—a foresighted but misunderstood pioneer in pursuit of a worthy goal.

Scientist

Maltz presents himself as a scientist engaged in discovering new techniques or refining old ones. He is no mere practitioner. Throughout his book, he provides detailed accounts of his operations in which he displays his virtuosity and inventiveness in repairing cleft palates, restoring deformed hands, or reconstructing noses. He always seems to be operating on his own—a solitary hero-surgeon, alone in his clinic in the sky (his clinic is situated in a penthouse on Fifth Avenue). If there is a nurse in attendance, we do not hear about her.

Maltz is supremely self-confident. Even when he uses an unfamiliar technique, he never doubts his abilities or that his plan of action is justified. As a scientist, he realizes that risks are part of the game, and he continually underlines the necessity of experimenting with new procedures. Plastic surgery is not a specialty for the timid or the conventional but requires qualities of daring and the willingness to embark on unknown paths. Already as an intern in Berlin, he admits to having had the "temerity to attempt to improve on the surgical instruments devised by the father of modern rhinoplasty, the Great Jacques Joseph himself" (17). Later, he provides a gripping account of one of his early operations with a skin graft. He knows that if the operation is unsuccessful, he will stand convicted as someone who had taken a chance and failed through lack of knowledge of what he was attempting to do and that "it would be hard to be more thoroughly blacklisted as a doctor" (67). However, with his faith in his new technique, he takes the risk:

> I was running with sweat and I should have been feeling tired, but I wasn't; I felt I had done very well; I felt that von Eicken would have been proud of me, and even Jacques Joseph; yes, I'd go beyond that—I felt that Harold Gillies [the originator of the skin graft procedure he was performing], had he been there, would have nodded in approval and told me that my modification of the Gillies tub was a clever piece of surgery. (64)

While his colleagues are in favor of the conservative approach (his superior warns that "the quickest way isn't necessarily the best"), Maltz situates himself as an enterprising man of science who is willing to take risks and to follow his intuitions even in the face of an uncertain outcome.[7]

Idealist

Maltz is not just a man of science; he is a man with a conscience as well. He presents himself as an idealistic physician who is, first and foremost, concerned with alleviating distress and helping people to live better lives. We are informed at the outset of the book that plastic surgery is a "very noble and compassionate form of the practice of medicine" (11), and this sentiment is repeated at regular intervals, particularly when Maltz is in danger of losing his faith in his profession. Interestingly, his idealism is most endangered by his female patients. Throughout the book, he makes disparaging remarks about these women as the "newly rich who are only interested in finding new

ways to spend their money" or "paper-millions ladies" who have discovered
that they can lose ten years with the simple, quick, and painless removal of
the crow's feet around the eyes or a "face-lift" (80).

Although Maltz enjoys the material advantages of his profession and is
clearly proud to have transcended his lowly origins, he makes it clear that
success has its price. It forces him into an ongoing struggle to sustain his idealistic vision about his profession. Whenever he feels particularly sickened by
the onslaught of wealthy society women seeking his services for trivial reasons, he begins to wonder whether he has lived up to his vision. Recalling his
experience as a young intern delivering a baby with a harelip in a tenement
building, he wonders whether the idealistic young man he was then would
consider that he had done well:

> God knows, in money, very well indeed. But was money what he had been
> thinking of, that windy, black morning as he stared at the pitiful little twisted
> face? The intern—and the boy out of whom he had grown—had been on famil-
> iar terms with the brawling, wrangling, rushing, day-in-and-day-out life of the
> city; down in the hot, dusty street, not aloft on the cool garden terraces, in the
> splendid room with the polite voices of fashionable patients. (145)

Maltz seeks redemption in patients with physical deformities ("a mis-
shapen face, scarred, burned, or harelipped") who are too poor to pay for his
services. He actively looks for them, overcomes their suspicions (often no
small task), and convinces them to let him help them, free of charge. The
neighborhood newspaper vendor with webbed hands, the kindly candy shop
owner from his old neighborhood with an unsightly scar, or the little girl
with the "ski-jump" nose are presented as examples of the recipients of
Maltz's altruism. By helping poor, working-class, and usually male patients, his commitment to his original ideals is reinstated. In this way, he
establishes himself as an idealist who is not simply motivated by fame and
financial success.[8]

Creator

Maltz describes his work as nothing less than "creating miracles": "I could
whisk new noses out of the air. . . . just about everything lay within the com-
pass of my magical powers" (209). There seems to be no deformity that he
cannot fix and his operations are invariably successful, fulfilling "every
man's [*sic*] divine right to look human" (145). Maltz's "magical powers" are,
by no means, limited to changing his patients' bodies, however. He not only
eliminated scars and repaired damage with skin grafts, but removed the
"deeper scars" as well—"the scars of the mind" (220).

Interestingly, much of this autobiography of a plastic surgeon is devoted to tales about people whom Maltz helps in ways that do not involve surgery. For example, when a beautiful woman wants an operation on her face, he resists her request, relying on a mysterious "sixth sense," which tells him that this is not her "real" problem. Rather than sending her away empty-handed, he intervenes in such a way that—as he puts it—he can bring the unhappy woman "back to life" (124).

The objects of Maltz's divine interventions do not always want to be helped, often because of their—as he assures us—thoroughly unfounded fears that the operation will be painful. In such cases, he brushes off their objections, promising them that he can solve their problems. In most cases, he does convince his patients to go along with him, but some remain adamant that they do not want his services. (Interestingly, these candidates are always poor in contrast to the rich "ladies" who he has to fend off in order to maintain his ideals.) Maltz tends to transform such cases into a moral tale: for example, the plain "spinster" with the "bird-like face" who rejects the possibility of becoming more beautiful as trivial compared to the delight she has in making children laugh (even when it is her face they are laughing at!).

Despite—or perhaps because of—his own God-like abilities to intervene in people's lives, Maltz presents himself as sensitive to the problem in others. For example, he describes catching his butler Rudolph surreptitiously trying on his white coat, trying to emulate him. Maltz invites him to an operation, taking great pleasure in his servant's fainting at the sight of blood. This moral lesson establishes Maltz sovereign power, while chastising his servant for getting "too big for his britches."[9]

Maltz's most sublime creation is presented in the final chapter when he (re)creates his lost love, Sylvia, by operating on her daughter and remaking her in the image of her mother. Reminiscent of Zeus bypassing the Mother Goddess Metis and giving birth to Athena from his head, Maltz incorporates the creativity of artist-surgeon with metaphorical fatherhood and the divine powers of a deity.[10] Plastic surgery enables him to gain a daughter and regain the woman he has lost. "There, looking at herself in the mirror, was another Sylvia; and though to be sure in only very small measure, in part she really was mine" (223). Sylvia belongs to Maltz in a way that was not possible before. By operating on her daughter, she becomes his—his creation.

Aesthete

Maltz presents himself as a lover of beauty, particularly in women. However, his relationship to beautiful women is ambivalent. Throughout his autobiography, he expresses a mixture of contempt and admiration for a particular class of women—the beautiful, wealthy "fur-clad" ladies who come to him for help. As a short, chubby, inexperienced youth from the Lower East Side, Maltz desired such women from a distance, realizing that they were firmly outside his reach. Writing about his first love, Sylvia, he contrasts her ("She was everything I wasn't. She, with her lovely face, her beautiful clear skin, her expensive clothes, her well-to-do family in New York, her careful schooling, her high-priced piano lessons") with his own situation, living in a "garret-coffin on the other, the very, very wrong side of Berlin" (21). Ultimately, Sylvia jilts him, and Maltz displaces his love for her onto the myriad women he meets in his practice as a plastic surgeon. Although he sometimes socializes with these patients, the encounters are also marked by contempt and rarely move beyond a platonic friendship.

Although he does occasionally encounter women who are interested in marrying him, he appears to have little interest in them. For example, when his mother attempts to matchmake him with a nice Jewish girl from the neighborhood ("a fine, safe and sane girl . . . who would watch the pennies and feed me well" and help him set up a "homely . . . practice such as Dr. Smargel's" [48]), he rejects her proposal on the grounds that it wouldn't work with a "queer fish" like himself. The "Judy Rinkers" of the world are not for someone who wants to become that "strange kind of doctor known as a plastic surgeon" (48). When he is middle-aged and successful, Maltz falls briefly in love with a patient after giving her a "face-lift." However, as soon as he receives a message from his old love, Sylvia, he abandons his would-be fiancée without further ado. Sylvia, of course, has no intention to returning to Maltz, so he is left, once again, alone with his fantasies of the ideal woman.

Drawing upon the Pygmalion myth of the sculptor who fell in love with his own creation and begs Venus to transform her into a woman, Maltz seems resigned to his fate, philosophically referring to the incident as the gods giving "a malicious twist to my elbow . . . so that Pygmalion would spoil his Galatea and fall out of love with her!" (194). Briefly saddened, he throws himself into his work. Ultimately, it is here that he finds a resolution of sorts for his problems with women. When he transforms Sylvia's daughter into the image of her mother, he has made her into his "statue"—not the "real thing," perhaps, but, nevertheless, a woman who is lovely enough for him to love.

Maltz idealizes women as beautiful objects and yet has difficulties with real women. He describes his patients as objects of art, to be admired from a distance. And, indeed, he seems to prefer the beauty of his creation to the "real thing." As soon as his Galatea becomes a woman, Maltz runs away or seeks solace in his work. Maltz's constant search for the ideal woman goes hand in hand with his craft; he can create a perfect woman while shunning relationships with women of flesh and blood.

In conclusion, Maxwell Maltz constructs himself as an enlightened pioneer, endowed with impressive technical skills and the mentality of a scientist who is unafraid to take risks for the greater good. Although he is successful, he remains an idealist. He is determined to help the physically deformed and damaged, whether or not they actually want to be helped. He is a creator with the skills to not only remake his patients' bodies, but also their lives. Endowed with an almost God-like omniscience that enables him to see through his patient's motives to the "real" problem beneath, Maltz is the ultimate creator: God in a white coat. And, finally, he is a lover of beautiful women who resolutely refuses to settle for anything short of perfection.

MASCULINE STORIES

Autobiographies are structured differently, depending on whether the author is a man or a woman (Gergen and Gergen 1993). Men's autobiographies typically concern a high-status or successful man in single-minded pursuit of his career. The protagonist generally has to do battle with opposing forces whereby he bravely tackles obstacles standing in the way of his goal. Men's autobiographies are about the "spirit defeating the flesh," whereby the protagonist displays bravado and self-assurance rather than giving way to self-doubt or feelings of vulnerability. Women's autobiographies, in contrast, weave together themes of achievement along with themes of love lives, children, and friendship. The female protagonist is likely to express her emotions, and women's stories are full of self-deprecation and uncertainty (196).

Doctor Pygmalion is a masculine story. It is a masculine story because the protagonist puts his career first. He has one goal and that is to become a successful plastic surgeon. His personal life is invariably subsumed under his career. Anecdotes about family or friends stand in relation to his career. His relationships with men are marked by competition and rivalry if they are powerful (his teachers, colleagues) and benevolent paternalism if they are not (his patients, his servant). If the hero is sometimes lonely or complains about not having a partner, this is, at best, a minor impediment to his well-being. Unlike a woman, he does not need relationships with other people in order to have a life that has made sense.

Doctor Pygmalion is a masculine story because it is structured as a typical heroic epic. The male protagonist has a quest, while the female is, at best, the object of this quest. As such, it resonates with American pioneer stories in which men seek adventure out west where danger and excitement await them. Women, of course, are the ones who stay behind, minding the hearth. When our hero Maltz rejects the safety of a neighborhood practice and the girl next door, he is simply enacting the story of the lonely cowboy riding out into the great unknown, more at ease with the uncertainties of the future than certainties of his past.

Doctor Pygmalion is a masculine story because it celebrates mind over matter, rationality over irrationality, and abstract values over concrete needs of specific individuals. Unlike women's autobiographies, which are oriented toward their own bodies and emotions (and the emotions of others), this protagonist is disembodied. If he feels discomfort about the situation in which he must do his work (Berlin) or the fact that he is unable to maintain a relationship with a woman, he simply blusters his way out of it. His morality is all encompassing and abstract ("noble and compassionate") but is singularly oblivious to the concrete particulars of his patients' lives, let alone to their own desires and needs. It is his ideals rather than the wishes of his patients that are at stake.

And, finally, *Doctor Pygmalion* is the masculine story because it expresses the contradictory and ambivalent relationship between masculinity and femininity. It draws upon—and, indeed, is named after—the myth of Pygmalion— a myth that constructs men as subjects and women as objects. This myth has a long and venerable history, has been recycled several times, but in each rendition remains a parable of the dilemmas of masculinity. The original Pygmalion was a king of Cypress who fell hopelessly in love with a statue of the beautiful Aphrodite. In his *Metamorphoses*, the Roman poet Ovid transformed the king into a sculptor with an aversion for women, who decides to create a statue of a woman more beautiful than any mortal woman could ever be. As fate would have it, this Pygmalion falls hopelessly—and obsessively[11]— in love with his own creation and prays to the gods to give him a woman like his ivory statue. Venus takes pity on him, Galatea awakes, and they live happily ever after.

Freud took up the Pygmalion myth in his analysis of a popular novella of his time: W. Jensen's *Gradiva*.[12] This is the story of a young archeologist who falls in love with a relief of a young Roman girl—or, more specifically, with her characteristic gait—and becomes so obsessed with her that he travels to Pompeii in search of her. Freud (1909) treats this as a case of obsessional delusion, referring to the fatal combination of repressed male sexual energy and the equally masculine fear of intimacy with a real woman (most notably, the archeologist's childhood sweetheart). The most familiar rendition of the myth, at least for modern readers, is George Bernard Shaw's play *Pygmalion*, written in 1916 (and adapted in 1956 as the popular musical *My Fair Lady*). This Pygmalion is a confirmed bachelor and woman hater, Henry Higgins. The artist has become a professor of linguistics, and his Galatea is the ignorant flower girl, Eliza, with a deplorable accent and working-class manners. Higgins decides to transform her into a lady with impeccable English.

What these renditions of the Pygmalion myth have in common is their portrayal of the "typical" male conflict between the desire for and fear of women. Feminist scholars have repeatedly linked masculinity—at least, in its white, Western, heterosexual forms—to men being socialized to suppress their identification with their mothers and to orient themselves to the unknown world of men outside the home (Chodorow 1978 and 1989; Hollway 1984; Flax 1990; Segal 1990). This separation is fragile, leaving men vulnerable and inclined to project their weaknesses or feelings of irrationality or dependence onto women. The crux of masculinity, then, is an ambivalence between longing for the unreachable woman (the mother) and a fear of femininity in one's self. Pygmalions enact this prototypical masculine story in their intellectual or artistic idealization of woman and their aversion toward or contempt for actual women. They can escape their own feelings and embodiment, by projecting them onto women. They become the disembodied and powerful creators, while women are the passive objects, inert clay waiting to be shaped according to the artist's intentions. Pygmalions can play out their fantasies of being God. As Bordo (1987) has argued, man has—even since the ancients—attempted to overcome the material exigencies of everyday life by associating the male with the mind, the soul, and divinity ("those qualities which the human shares with God" [94]) and disassociating himself with all that is material, embodied, and female.

But the Pygmalion myth expresses the contradictions of masculinity as well. While Ovid's hero escapes with some help from Venus, latter-day Pygmalions have had to go it alone, remaining locked in their masculine obsessions and ambivalent relationships with femininity. Shaw's Pygmalion, Professor Higgins, merely shrugs his shoulders when his Eliza leaves him to marry another man; Freud's protagonist prefers his hopeless love of an image of an ancient beauty, Gradiva, to his childhood sweetheart; and Maxwell Maltz—he continues to operate.

MASCULINITY AND MEDICINE

Doctor Pygmalion is not simply the particularized story of one man's life. It is the story of a profession. Maltz consistently presents himself as the mouthpiece of this profession, as the person whose task it is to set out the wonders of the "noble and compassionate" practice of plastic surgery. His "personal story" is, therefore, not so personal at all. It expresses and is shaped by the discourses that are part of his profession—the profession of plastic surgery.

Since Foucault, we can appreciate the significance of discourses for understanding the origins and nature of institutional and clinical practices. Medical knowledge is not simply constituted by the human subject but shaped by the discursive formations of the historical, cultural, and social context in which it is produced. Just as Foucault could describe the emergence of the prison (1979) or the clinic (1973 and 1975) through the accounts of prison directors or physicians, Maltz's autobiography provides evidence of the kinds of discourses that shaped the practices of the emerging profession of plastic surgery.

The medical system is gendered, at the level of interaction between practitioners and patients, in the organization of its institution and practices, and in the conflation of its discourses with symbolic notions of masculinity and femininity. Historically, medicine emerged in the wake of a male-initiated takeover of women's control over healing and other matters related to reproduction like sexuality, birth, spirituality, and death (Ehrenreich and English 1979; Hearn 1987). Although the profession of medicine has since opened its doors to women, it still remains an indisputably male preserve. Gender segregation and exclusion of women from the higher echelons of medicine go hand in hand with powerful medical discourses that construct women as archetypical patients: diseased, neurotic, and in need of repair (Ehrenreich and English 1979; Martin 1987; Jacobus et al. 1990). In contrast, men are viewed as imminently suited to the job of physician, while male patients are rendered invisible.[13] Medical professionality draws upon a gendered dichotomy between rationality and emotionality, whereby the patient is tied to the life world through her emotions and her body while the practitioner may escape his emotions and body by maintaining a veneer of objectivity and "gentlemanly reasonableness" (Hearn 1987; Davis 1988). Rationality, objectivity, and instrumentality are the hallmarks of medical science and masculinity. The image of science as quest for discovery and control over the unruly forces of nature runs through modern science from Plato to the present (Keller 1983). The male scientist is presented as the rational, disembodied mind while the object of his ministrations displays all features that are associated with femininity: irrationality, nature, and the body.

Plastic surgery is a quintessentially masculine profession or, to paraphrase David Morgan (1981), an example of masculinity in medical robes. Plastic surgery produces and reproduces masculinity as an integral feature of the historical, cultural, and institutional practices and discourses of medicine. It reflects the gendered imbalances of medicine in its high incidence of male practitioners as well as its overrepresentation of women among its patients. It draws upon discourses of gender in its deployment of images of the physician as God-like creator rather than healer, in its tendency to privilege adventure over the mundane and everyday and in its idealization of feminine beauty (or woman with a W), while rendering ordinary women ugly, deficient, and in need of improvement (Young 1990a).

In conclusion, *Doctor Pygmalion* enables us to understand why the profession of plastic surgery might be particularly attractive to male surgeons, while proving impenetrable territory for women as surgeons. It not only offers ample possibilities for the expression of masculinity—as lonely cowboys, as scientific heroes, or as God-like creator. It also provides a particularly compelling expression of and resolution to masculine fears of femininity, enabling the practitioner to idealize femininity while avoiding real, flesh-and-blood women.

NOTES

I would like to thank Willem de Haan, Lena Inowlocki, Nora Räthzel, José van Dyck, and Dubravka Zarkov for their helpful and insightful comments.

1. See *Plastic Surgery Information Service,* Expanded Version 2001 Statistics.

2. Within the profession of plastic surgery, a distinction is made between "reconstructive" and "cosmetic" or "aesthetic" surgery. "Reconstructive" is generally used for surgery that restores function, while "cosmetic" refers to procedures that are regarded as medically unnecessary or "just for looks." While the distinction is blurry in practice, it has historically been the subject of ongoing strife within the organization concerning which kind of surgery was appropriately "medical" and which was the domain of charlatans or quacks. "Cosmetic surgery" is a more recent and probably the most popular designation for surgery intended to improve or preserve attractiveness (see Gilman 1999, 8–16).

3. This might be compared to other autobiographies, which show the author at different stages in his or her life, family members and colleagues, places of residence or employment.

4. While several well-known plastic surgeons were operating in the United States by the time Maltz became interested, the training programs did not allow students the experience of actually cutting up corpses—a practice that was permitted in Germany.

5. Following World War II, the Veterans Administration organized a spate of "quickie courses" for physicians, designed to teach them the techniques of plastic surgery within two to three days (McDowell 1985). It seems likely that Maltz's trips to VA hospitals fall under that heading. While he presents this activity as a sign that he has arrived as an expert in his field, McDowell refers to it as a "sordid chapter" in the history of plastic surgery, where established surgeons profited from their less successful colleagues and, at the same time, enabled poorly trained practitioners to engage in plastic surgery.

6. Although plastic surgery is one of the oldest medical interventions, it maintains an image of a nascent specialty. Contemporary plastic surgeons tend to discuss their field as still having to fight prejudice in order to be accepted as a full-fledged medical specialty.

7. This feature can be found in many biographies of famous scientists whose lives are presented as adventure stories in which the protagonist rejects the role of "dull lab worker" in favor of the solitary genius who stubbornly and sometimes arrogantly crosses his friends and colleagues in order to chart new horizons (Van Dijck 1997).

8. Contemporary plastic surgeons are also compelled to upgrade the image of their profession. Particularly in view of the enormous cosmetic surgery "craze" in recent years, surgeons are often suspected (and probably correctly) of operating with an eye to profit. Moreover, they run the risk of being viewed as spending their time indulging their primarily female clientele's trivial desire for beauty rather than helping patients who are suffering from "real" problems. Like Maltz, these surgeons often justify their work with references to their altruistic motives and their work with "deserving" patients—usually men with industrial injuries or children suffering from burns or congenital birth defects.

9. Interestingly, most of Maltz's relationships with other men—his teacher and colleagues, his servants, Sylvia's husband—are fraught with competition. The only exceptions are his male, usually working-class patients.

10. Wilshire (1989) provides an interesting discussion of the use of god (and goddess) mythology in the discourses of modern science. The image of Zeus disassociating himself from the lowliness of the body and its matter, including his own infancy and mother, and giving birth out of his head represents the male disembodied mind, while women remain tied to their material bodies and unruly emotions and are, therefore, unsuited for scientific endeavors.

11. Ovid describes how the sculptor can't stop touching, caressing, and kissing his ivory statue. He begins to dress her and adorn her with jewels, presenting her with small presents (canary birds, fruit). Ultimately, he places her on a divan in a reclining position, with cushions under her head (Ovid 1993, 243–97).

12. I would like to thank Janet Sayers for drawing my attention to this case study.

13. While contemporary plastic surgeons are prone to making statements about the increase in surgery among men, implying that equality has arrived in matters of appearance, they are notably reticent to elaborate on the particulars of men's difficulties with their appearance.

3

The Rhetoric of Cosmetic Surgery: Luxury or Welfare

Medical interventions in the human body are burgeoning. From open-heart surgery to organ transplants to gene therapy and the new reproductive technologies, the possibilities for technological enhancement seem almost unlimited. While these interventions are supposed to prolong life, improve health, or enhance well-being, in practice, they are often dangerous, expensive, and morally problematic. In recent years, controversies have emerged about the desirability of such extensive medical meddling in the human body and life cycle. One such controversy concerns cosmetic surgery, which is by far the fastest growing medical specialty, both in the United States and abroad. Millions of people—most of whom are women—flock to plastic surgeons each year to have their faces "lifted," their breasts "enhanced," or their tummies "tucked," as the operations are euphemistically called. It has been estimated that more than two million Americans undergo some form of cosmetic surgery every year.[1]

Despite the enormous popularity of cosmetic surgery, the operations are invariably painful; have myriad, often permanent side effects;[2] and frequently leave the recipient in worse shape than she was before the operation. Feminists have been unanimously critical of cosmetic surgery as a practice, which reproduces ideologies of sexual inferiority instructing women that their bodies are not good enough: too fat, too flat chested, too old, or too "ethnic." Cosmetic surgery is regarded—and rightly so—as a particularly pernicious expression of the disciplinary regimes of the feminine beauty system—as a way, quite literally, to "cut women down to size."

Cosmetic surgery is not only controversial for feminists, however. The medical profession has increasingly found itself in the position of having to

59

justify performing dangerous surgical interventions on otherwise healthy bodies. Moreover, in the wake of a rapidly aging population and the state's inability to meet even basic health care needs, medical insurance companies have to warrant funding expensive operations for what is often seen as a luxury problem. The medical sociologist Nora Jacobson (2000) has provided an excellent history of breast implant technology in the United States in which she pays special attention to the controversies that have emerged concerning the safety of implant devices. She shows how the meanings surrounding breast implants were shaped by plastic surgeons, implant manufacturers, the Food and Drug Administration, the media, and consumer groups in ways that have led both to the acceptance but also to the refusal of implants. Breast implants have been treated at different times and in different contexts as "unnatural" foreign bodies, as treatment for women suffering from the pathological condition of "flat chestedness"—and as an aide for psychologically healthy women with an honest desire to "feel better about themselves" (Jacobson 2000, 120).

In this chapter, I want to explore some of the debates that have emerged in the Netherlands concerning cosmetic surgery. The Netherlands is an interesting case because it has the somewhat dubious distinction of being the only country in the world to actually have included cosmetic surgery in its basic health care package. Any individual who could demonstrate that she or he needed cosmetic surgery could have it paid for by national health insurance. As a result, more cosmetic surgery was performed per capita in the Netherlands than in the United States.[3] This cosmetic surgery "boom" was, financially speaking, bad news for a welfare system that was already having difficulties meeting even the most basic health care needs of its rapidly aging population. Cuts had to be made, and cosmetic surgery, along with other medical practices, became the subject of heated debate. Was it necessary for the welfare of a particular individual, or was it a luxury item that did not belong in the basic health care package?

Based on the problems that emerged in trying to justify cosmetic surgery in the Netherlands, as well as the outcome of the debate, I will discuss some of the limitations of a moral rhetoric based on equality, universality, and distributive justice for defending cosmetic surgery—and, by implication, other controversial medical practices like in vitro fertilization (IVF), gene therapy, and "smart drugs." This having been done, I want to argue that an ethic that draws upon a rhetoric of difference, particularity, and need can provide a better starting point for coming to terms with the ethical issues that these practices raise.

THE RHETORIC OF HEALTH CARE

In different health care systems, different rhetorical strategies are drawn upon to justify, defend, or criticize controversial medical technologies and practices. As David Frankford (1998) has convincingly argued, health care policy is not based on the incontrovertible facts of the case. It is a social process by which actors "grab" their arguments from justificatory frameworks available to them and deploy these arguments in such a way that they will resonate with what has already been constituted as feasible, reasonable, and desirable.

Policy is not the rational connection of ends to means, the properly calibrated choice of inducements, rules, rights, and penalties, but rather consists in the rhetorical making of a case—the statement of what is and what ought to be (Frankford 1998, 73–74). The rhetoric used in such debates depends, among other things, upon the way health care is organized.

In a market system, like the United States, health care is provided on a fee-for-service basis, and medical services tend to be distributed on the basis of availability. Specialists are "free" to provide services, just as patients are "free" to choose the health care they desire, provided they can pay for it. In principle, patients are consumers with equal rights to health care. In practice, public access is not guaranteed, and many services are, therefore, only available to the affluent.

In a market system, the rhetoric used to justify controversial medical practices and technologies revolves around the issues of risk, malpractice, and informed consent. The medical profession, and, more indirectly, the regulatory bureaucracy are accountable for practicing medicine in such a way that risks are kept at a minimum. Patients are free to use dangerous or experimental medical procedures, provided they know what they are getting into. This having been done, patients are left to "choose" for themselves.

In a welfare system, like the Netherlands and most Western European countries, health care is provided by the state, and medical services are distributed on the basis of necessity. In principle, a patient has a right to any form of health care he or she needs. Health care is not simply a privilege to be enjoyed by those who can afford it, but an entitlement for every citizen, regardless of his or her social position. In practice, however, many services are too expensive for the state to fund. The most common dilemma in the European welfare model of medicine is the increasingly articulated need for particular services and technologies and the equally pressing necessity to limit government expenditure on health care.

In a welfare system, the rhetoric used to justify medical practices and technologies revolves around issues of welfare versus luxury and how to make choices in heath care. The medical profession shares at least some of the responsibility for the overall expense of the health care system. The main focus of medical accountability is whether a particular practice or technology is a luxury or really necessary for citizens' health and well-being. A discourse of need shifts attention from risk to whether a particular medical service or procedure is "really" necessary in a context of scarcity. There is generally an implicit or explicit consensus that "unnecessary" services cannot be included in the basic health care package and must, therefore, be abandoned or made available through other means.

An example is the "Choices in Care" debate in the Netherlands. This was a broad, government-sponsored campaign to convince Dutch citizens of the necessity of making decisions about the availability of medical procedures, technologies, and medications. A governmental task force—the Dunning Commission—was established to develop normative criteria for evaluating health care services (Ministry of Health, Education, and Welfare 1992).[4] They came up with the following guidelines for making assessments: Is the service necessary? Is it effective? Does it do what it is intended to do? Could the service be provided through private means? It was assumed that by evaluating the health care services currently covered by national health insurance, services could be removed from the basic health care package, thereby reducing health care expenditure.

I shall now turn to the actual debate on cosmetic surgery in the Netherlands.

THE DUTCH CASE

Prior to 1980, cosmetic surgery was a small, but acceptable, branch of plastic surgery in the Netherlands. Like any other medical practice, it was included in the basic health care package, provided the surgeon thought it was necessary. Initially, plastic surgeons did not justify performing cosmetic surgery in terms of the patient's physical characteristics. Instead, they claimed that a deficient appearance was a source of psychosocial problems and could cause an unacceptable degree of damage to the person's happiness and well-being. They defended cosmetic surgery patients against charges of vanity or hypochondria. On the contrary, they argued, there were many sound "psychological" reasons for wanting surgery: bereavement (and wanting to find a new partner), feelings of inferiority, sexual frigidity, and more. Children with "jug ears" ran the risk of being teased by their classmates, and women with sagging breasts were afraid to go swimming in public pools or undress in dressing rooms. Problems with appearance could easily lead to antisocial or even suicidal behavior. Cosmetic surgery was, therefore, not a *luxury,* but a *necessity* for alleviating a specific kind of problem. The term "welfare surgery" was born (Bouman 1975).[5]

Cosmetic surgery became problematic, however, when, in the early eighties, there was a dramatic increase in cosmetic surgery with nearly every type of operation doubling in frequency (Starmans 1988). For a welfare state already in crisis, this expansion was bad news. In an attempt to stem the flow of applicants for cosmetic surgery, plastic surgeons, together with the medical inspectors from the national health insurance companies, were asked to develop guidelines for making decisions about which operations were necessary and which were not. They began by establishing three categories of cosmetic surgery that would be eligible for coverage by national health insurance:

- a functional disturbance or affliction (for example, eyelids that droop to such an extent that vision is impaired)
- severe psychological suffering (the patient is under psychiatric treatment specifically for problems with appearance)
- a physical imperfection that falls outside a "normal degree of variation in appearance" (the patient's appearance does not meet certain aesthetic standards as determined by the medical inspector)

The first two categories were unproblematic as the criteria could be derived within medical discourse. Moreover, patients rarely applied for cosmetic surgery due to severe psychological suffering because it meant bringing a report from a psychiatrist. The majority of the cosmetic surgery recipients fell under the third category, and it was this category—"outside a normal variation in appearance"—that proved to be something of a headache for the national health insurance system and, indirectly, for the plastic surgeons.

Initially, medical experts, in collaboration with the national health insurance system, attempted to develop guidelines for abnormal appearance. They looked for criteria that could be objectively observed, classified, and applied to all candidates for cosmetic surgery. Undeterred by the adage that "beauty is in the eye of the beholder," they originally seemed convinced that appearance—just like any other feature of the body—could be assessed scientifically.

Some problems did, indeed, seem to be amenable to classification. For example, ears could be measured in centimeters; that is, how far they protruded from the side of the head. Other problems received more praxeological criteria. For example, a breast lift was indicated if the "nipples were level with the recipient's elbows." A "difference of four clothing sizes between top and bottom" was sufficient indication that a breast augmentation or liposuction were in order. Although these criteria may not sound exactly scientific, they did have the advantage of being clear-cut. Other criteria were much more vague. For example, for a face-lift, the person's countenance should look "ten years older than her or his chronological age." A sagging abdomen that "makes her look pregnant" provided reason enough for performing an abdominoplasty ("tummy tuck"). Eyelid corrections were justified if "the person looks like he or she has been out drinking all evening."

Such were the criteria that were developed in order to decide "objectively" whether or not an operation was necessary and, therefore, deserved full medical coverage. The fact that they seemed to be based more on common sense than science is only part of the problem. More seriously, they proved totally inadequate in the practical context of having to decide which kinds of cosmetic surgery should be covered by national health insurance. Let me illustrate this with an example concerning a relatively minor form of cosmetic surgery: the removal of tattoos.

Initially, it was agreed that tattoo removal should not be covered by national health insurance. The argument was that tattoos are put on voluntarily at the recipient's own expense and should, therefore, be taken off in the same way. This seemed fairly straightforward until a large number of Moroccan immigrant women began coming in to have their tattoos removed. The medical inspectors began to falter, wondering—as they put it—just how voluntary the tattoos of these women had actually been. Whereas tattooing in Holland was apparently considered a part of the individual's right to experiment with her or his body, tattooing in Morocco was viewed as a practice performed under coercion—a symbol of cultural constraint. The reasoning was that if such tattoos had not been done voluntarily and were, furthermore, detrimental to migrant women's integration into Dutch society and, by implication, her well-being, then an exception had to be made. Thus, the criterion was changed: surgical removal of tattoos was covered by national health, provided the recipient was not Dutch born.

No sooner had this new guideline been established, when the next problem arose in the form of a highly publicized rape case in which the rapist had drugged his victim and tattooed his name on her stomach. When she came in to have the name of her assailant removed surgically, she was denied coverage on the grounds that she was Dutch born. The victim filed a complaint, and the press got hold of the incident, much to the embarrassment of the medical inspectors. After several behind-closed-door meetings, national health decided that, once again, an exception should be made.

The tattoo episode is but one example of the complexities surrounding cosmetic surgery. However, it highlights the ethical dilemmas facing the medical profession in deciding when and where cosmetic surgery was necessary and when it was not. In the course of repeated confrontations with exceptional cases, the medical profession was continually forced to go beyond its own discourse and draw upon subjective or commonsensical arguments or, more problematically, the available ideological discourses. This meant—at least in the Netherlands—liberal individualism and ethnocentrism.

All attempts to develop general rules for applying guidelines to particular cases failed in the face of the myriad exceptions. Medical inspectors for the national health insurance companies openly complained about having to make practical decisions on coverage without having adequate guidelines. And, more seriously, after nearly a decade of trying to get the expansion of cosmetic surgery under control, the number of operations showed no signs of abating.

The medical experts and welfare bureaucrats began to concede that making decisions about who should have cosmetic surgery was a hopelessly subjective enterprise. A short, heated, and somewhat belated public debate ensued. Several plastic surgeons wrote impassioned pieces in the local newspapers defending cosmetic surgery as essential for their patients' well-being. However, these proponents of cosmetic surgery as "welfare surgery" were ultimately overruled. Since the medical profession was unable to back up the welfare argument with a plan for stemming the flow of operations, there was no other recourse but to hand it over to the national health insurance companies. Although cosmetic surgery could have easily and, indeed, effectively been assessed according to the four criteria recommended by the Dunning Commission, the Council for the National Health Insurance System decided to make an exception in the case of cosmetic surgery and not to apply the usual criteria of necessity, effectiveness, functionality, and financial need. Instead they opted to eliminate cosmetic surgery without further discussion from the basic health care package. Coverage was subsequently limited to those few cases that could be justified unproblematically in medical discourse—that is, through a functional or psychiatric disturbance. The solution to the problem of cosmetic surgery was, therefore, to drop the welfare argument and leave cosmetic surgery for strictly aesthetic reasons to the private sector. This move met with little protest from a public that had already tended to see cosmetic surgery as a somewhat trivial intervention—"something for middle-aged ladies with nothing better to do."[6]

Recent developments show how shortsighted this ruling was. Since 1991, the number of individuals seeking psychiatric treatment for reasons of appearance has doubled. More than half of all patients contesting decisions concerning national health coverage are applicants for some form of cosmetic surgery. The majority of these appeals are denied, and, interestingly, this is done in one of two ways. One way is to argue that the applicant's psychological problems are not serious enough to warrant a surgical solution ("who doesn't have trouble with her appearance?"). The other is to claim that the applicant's problems are so extensive that cosmetic surgery will not make a difference ("that patient has so much wrong with her that a nip or a tuck is not going to help"). This damned-if-you-do-and-damned-if-you-don't line of reasoning provides a rather chilling indication of the unwillingness on the part of the medical profession and the welfare bureaucrats to take the suffering of cosmetic surgery candidates seriously.

The Dutch case illustrates some of the shortcomings of a discourse of equality, universalism, and distributive justice in the context of a welfare system of health care with limited resources. It shows the drawbacks of an approach that does not place the demand for a particular medical service in a broader social context where specific groups are differentially involved—either because they express different needs for medical intervention or because the medical profession is more inclined to dispense certain forms of health care to specific groups. It also shows the limitations of an approach that tries to make choices in care and, therefore, to cut costs according to general guidelines that are equally applicable to all patients. Applying general rules indiscriminately to individual cases cannot do justice in cases where there are special circumstances or special needs. And, it shows that the job of cutting costs and making choices cannot and should not be left to the medical profession. It highlights the impossibility of making just choices and defending necessary cutback operations without the participation of patients and other concerned parties.

ETHICAL GUIDELINES

In *Reshaping the Female Body* (1995), I developed a framework that enabled me to critically situate cosmetic surgery in a broader social, cultural, and political context, while, at the same time, to find a way to justify it as a solution for problems of suffering in special cases. This required a kind of balancing act: finding a way to be critical of the practice, which is dangerous, demeaning, or oppressive, without uncritically undermining the recipients—most of whom are women—who see it as their best and, in some cases, only option for alleviating suffering that has gone beyond the point of endurance.

The same balancing act may well be required of the medical profession and welfare bureaucracy, if they want to take the needs of the individual seriously as well as acknowledge the inevitable limitations of a welfare system where choices in care have to be made. In thinking about ethical guidelines for dealing with controversial medical practices more adequately, I have looked to contemporary feminist ethics for inspiration. Drawing on the work of several feminist philosophers—Iris Marion Young (1990a), Seyla Benhabib (1992), and Nancy Fraser (1989)—I will make a modest proposal for a critical assessment of cosmetic surgery in public debates based on a politics of difference, particularity, and need.

Difference

My first ethical guideline would require a critical stance toward any argument for or against cosmetic surgery, which does not take into account differences associated with gender, social class, ethnicity or religion, sexual preference, or age. Most welfare policy is based on the idea that people are basically the same in terms of their health care needs. However, group differences are often implicated in an individual's bodily experiences, sense of well-being, chances of becoming ill, and the kinds of services she or he seeks. It makes no sense to talk about medical interventions like cosmetic surgery as gender-neutral or nonracialized practices. In the Netherlands, for example, a Moroccan immigrant woman may have difficulties experiencing her facial tattoos as "just" a body adornment, comparable to practices like ear piercing or hair dyeing. Her tattoos mark her as "Other"—downtrodden and tied to the past. Even if her reasons for having them removed seem familiar (she's tired of looking at them in the mirror every morning; she just wants a change), she will do well to present her desire for surgery as culturally motivated so that the surgeon can "rescue" her from the clutches of her backward culture and help her become assimilated in Dutch society.[7]

Iris Young (1990a) has elaborated this process under the term "aesthetic scaling of bodies" as one of the ways privileged groups—notably white, Western, professional men—transcend their own material bodies and take a God's eye view as disembodied subjects. They are the ones who set the standards and judge, rather than the ones who are judged against standards they can never hope to meet. The process of body scaling takes place in everyday interactive contexts and within cultural discourses, whereby groups falling outside the dominant standard of appearance are devalued. This kind of inferiorization works at the level of practical consciousness where it is difficult to change precisely because it falls outside what is discursively available to both the assessor as well as the object of his or her assessment. In Young's view, being unaware of what one is doing does not excuse a person from making these unconscious areas explicit and amenable to public discussion, and she, therefore, holds dominant groups responsible for their "gut level" responses, including ethnocentrism and processes of "othering." She advocates a politics of difference, which takes issue with the abstract, universalized notions of the "individual" in relation to an equally abstract notion of "policy," and focuses instead on specific histories of inferiorization. Such a politics would aim at understanding why certain bodies in certain contexts are defined as deficient and in need of change. It would also enable an analysis of why interventions like cosmetic surgery might seem acceptable or desirable in some cases, but unacceptable or even repugnant in others.[8]

Particularity

My second ethical guideline would entail a critical stance toward any definitive argument for or against cosmetic surgery, which makes it impossible to
consider the particularities of the individual recipient. Particularities are essential for understanding when an individual's suffering has gone beyond an
acceptable limit. Most welfare policy ignores the subjective and local experience of particular individuals and, consequently, tends to turn a blind eye to
suffering that falls outside the standard provisions for health care. The Dutch
case was an exception precisely because surgeons, the heath inspector for national health insurance, and various welfare policy makers spent many years
agonizing over which cases of cosmetic surgery should be covered by insurance and which should not. While this did not lead to unproblematic criteria,
as we have seen, it did increase the awareness within the medical profession
that cosmetic surgery could not be treated as a strictly medical matter. It was,
in fact, one of the few cases where surgeons were aware—often painfully
so—of the limitations of their practices. Moreover, they were compelled to
confront the normative dimensions of their decisions and to engage in public
debates about the ethics of cosmetic surgery. From time to time, they even
had a bad conscience, as the tattoo example attests.

The case of cosmetic surgery illustrates that, while there may be no objec-
tive criteria for *normal* appearance, in some cases suffering may well go beyond what a person should *normally* have to bear. Seyla Benhabib (1992) has
developed a conception of interactive dialogue, which joins respect for the
other person's story—the lived experiences, the individual misfortunes, the biographical circumstances—with procedures, which are open and fair to all.
She suggests that the goal of such a dialogue is not necessarily consensus or
unanimity, but "reaching an agreement" (9). In the case of cosmetic surgery,
if we are interested in minimizing pain that exceeds an acceptable limit, it is
clear that exceptions will always have to be made. Thus, an ethical guideline
is in order that takes the respect for the other's point of view—a willingness
to reason from his or her perspective—in a context where decisions have to
be made as a moral precept for finding ways to deal with the ubiquitous special case. This means being able to break rules as well as to make them.

Need

My third ethical guideline would require abandoning any argument that reduces choices in whether to fund health care services like cosmetic surgery
to distributive justice; that is, dispensing available services equally among
persons who are equally eligible to receive them. Most welfare policy is not

developed in a context of participation and debate and, consequently, does not encourage citizens to take responsibility for the kinds of choices that have to be made in a welfare system. However, a just health care system would depend upon its citizens' willingness to support the choices and shoulder the burden of the costs. The Dutch "Choices in Care" debate is, again, a case in point. Despite paying lip service to the importance of public discussion, the problem of cosmetic surgery was resolved behind doors, through a combination of medicalization and privatization. Appearance became a medical problem, and cosmetic surgery was left to the individual who could afford it. For most people, this strategy met with little opposition since they already believed that cosmetic surgery did not belong in the same league as open-heart surgery or home help for the chronically ill. For the recipients, it simply meant having to find a psychiatrist willing to verify that their problems were serious enough to warrant surgery or, should that fail, skipping a vacation in order to afford a trip to a private clinic. However, the Dutch "solution" was problematic in that it absolved the Dutch public from the bothersome task of having to wonder why some of its citizens might feel that they could not live with their bodies. There was no longer a need to entertain the uncomfortable possibility that something was amiss with Dutch culture if cosmetic surgery was the only avenue for some individuals to a "normal" life. And, finally, the dangers and risks of the operations as well as the question of whether certain technologies should be developed at all was reduced to a matter of individual risk assessment rather than treated as a matter of concern for the general public.[9]

I do not pretend that there is an easy solution to the problem of funding, and, perhaps, when all is said and done, cosmetic surgery should be taken out of a basic health care package. However, the "when all is said and done" should not be neglected. In this context, the political theorist Nancy Fraser (1989) has provided a useful alternative to distributive models for welfare services, which she calls a politics of need interpretation. Her assumption is that needs are always contradictory, multivalent, and contested. The "need" for cosmetic surgery is no exception. It is neither inherently beneficial or destructive, emancipatory or repressive, but requires an ongoing process of interpretation and contestation. Whether cosmetic surgery is "really" necessary should ideally be sorted out in a democratic, public discussion, involving different parties (recipients, patient organizations, policy makers, medical professionals, cultural critics). Whatever the outcome of this process, it will be a decision that does not deny the suffering of the individual, while, at the same time, ensuring that the public is confronted with the necessity of making difficult choices and being prepared to shoulder the burden of the special case.

CONCLUSION

In this chapter, I have presented a special case in a specific health care system at a specific stage of development. However, as I mentioned at the outset, I believe that this special case raises a number of questions that have a wider relevance, especially for those who would like to see the U.S. health care system develop in the direction of a welfare model. While it is not my intention to play down the advantages of this model, it behooves us all to realize that a welfare system has its difficulties as well, the most notable being that the time invariably comes where everything does not go as expected and hard choices need to be made. In that context, questions arise about what constitutes a necessary level of welfare and what should be protected by a basic health care plan and how to make health care services available in special cases, when necessary.

Answering these questions requires an ethic that prohibits both a blanket acceptance as well as a straightforward rejection of medical practices and technologies for prolonging life and enhancing the human body. An ethic is needed that enables us to acknowledge difference, to consider the "exceptional case," and to engage in a public process of need interpretation. Such an ethic would not eliminate the necessity of having to make choices in health care. Indeed, it would help us to make them.

NOTES

1. It is notoriously difficult to obtain accurate statistics on the actual numbers of operations performed. In both the United States and Europe, statistics are recorded for operations performed in hospitals by registered plastic surgeons. Since the majority of these operations are performed in private clinics, and many operations are not performed by plastic surgeons, such estimates do not begin to cover the actual incidence of cosmetic surgery. While there is also a "gray area" in U.S. statistics on cosmetic surgery, the American Society of Plastic Surgeons (ASPS) keeps records of the number and type of cosmetic surgery procedures performed each year as well as information on the sex, ethnicity, and age of the patients, and makes this available on the Internet. In the following chapters of this book, I will be drawing upon these figures.

2. Even the most minor interventions cause discomfort, ranging from the dead crust of skin left by a chemical peel to the swelling and inflammation of a face-lift. Other operations like abdominoplasties, breast corrections, and liposuctions fall under the category of major surgery, requiring hospitalization and sometimes intensive care. The list of side effects, some permanent, accompanying cosmetic surgery operations is long: infections, wound disruption, scar tissue, pain, numbness, bruising,

or discoloration of the skin. More serious disabilities include fat embolisms, blood clots, fluid depletion, damage to the immune system, and, in some cases, death. See Davis (1995).

3. The official estimate was 6,060 cosmetic surgery operations between 1980 and 1989, of which 5,925 were women (more than 97 percent). However, since there are thirty-nine private institutes in the Netherlands performing cosmetic surgery, the actual number of operations is considerably higher. National health experts have suggested that 20,000 might be a "modest estimate"; that is, nearly four times higher than the official figure!

4. The final report was translated into English and used as an example for Hillary Clinton's project to reform the American health care system.

5. This is similar to arguments made in the United States. See, for example, Haiken (1997) and Gilman (1998 and 1999).

6. As we saw in chapter 2, the tendency to trivialize people's reasons for having cosmetic surgery has a long history, both within and outside the medical profession.

7. In the course of my earlier research, I had the opportunity to observe how applicants for coverage for cosmetic surgery competently drew upon the cultural discourses at their disposal to persuade the health inspector that they should have the surgery. For example, one candidate of Surinamese descent claimed that she needed an abdominoplasty because all the women in her family were fat. "It's all the rice we eat."

8. I will be returning to this point in more detail in chapter 5.

9. A case in point is the silicone breast implant controversy in the United States. When news hit the Netherlands, the undersecretary of the health department announced that he saw no reason to take action as he was sure that "our surgeons had informed their patients about any possible risks" (*Volkskrant*, February 24, 1992). Apparently, if women were still determined to have their breasts enlarged, it was their own decision to take the risk.

4

Surgical Stories: Constructing the Body, Constructing the Self

Cosmetic surgery belongs to the growing arsenal of techniques and technologies for body improvement and beautification, which are part of the cultural landscape of late modernity. Women, who are numerically and ideologically the primary objects of these practices, have a long tradition of enduring pain "for the sake of beauty." From the practices of foot binding in ancient China to chemical face peeling and collagen-inflated lips in Southern California, women have been prepared to go to great lengths to meet cultural ideals of feminine shape and countenance.

The recent cosmetic surgery craze seems to be just one more expression—albeit a particularly dramatic and dangerous one—of what has been called the "feminine beauty system" (MacCannell and MacCannell 1987). This system includes an enormous complex of cultural beauty practices drawn upon by individual women in order to meet the contemporary requirements of feminine appearance. It is one of the central ways that Western femininity is produced and regulated.

Feminist scholars have tended to cast a critical eye on women's involvement with "the beauty system" (Wolf 1991). Originally, beauty was described in terms of suffering and oppression. Women were presented as the victims of beauty norms and of the ideology of feminine inferiority that they sustain. The beauty system was compared to the "military-industrial complex" and decried as a "major articulation of capitalist patriarchy" (Bartky 1990, 39–40). By linking the beauty practices of individual women to the structural constraints of the beauty system, a convincing case was made for treating beauty as an essential ingredient of the social subordination of women—an ideal way to keep women in line by lulling them into believing that they could gain control over their lives through continued vigilance over their bodies.

In recent years, feminist discourses on beauty as oppression have begun to make way for postmodern perspectives that treat beauty in terms of cultural discourses. The body remains a central concern, this time, however, as a text upon which culture writes its meanings. Following Foucault, the female body is portrayed as an "imaginary site," always available to be inscribed with meanings. It is here that femininity in all her diversity can be constructed— through scientific discourses, medical technologies, the popular media, and everyday common sense. In this framework, routine beauty practices belong to the disciplinary and normalizing regime of body improvement and trans- formation. They are part and parcel of the production of "docile bodies" (Fou- cault 1980). The postmodern shift in some contemporary forms of feminist theory enables a sensitivity to the multiplicity of meanings surrounding the female body as well as to the insidious workings of power in and through cul- tural discourses on beauty and femininity.

If feminists have had reason to be skeptical of the more mundane practices of the beauty system, it is not surprising that they are even more critical of the practice of cosmetic surgery. Cosmetic surgery goes beyond the more routine procedures of body improvement and maintenance, such as leg waxing, makeup, and dieting. Along with the pain and costs, it often involves serious side effects and the not-infrequent chance of permanent maiming, should the operation fail to achieve the desired result. With its expanding arsenal of techniques for reshaping and remaking the body, cosmetic surgery seems to be the site par excellence for disciplining and normalizing the female body— for, literally, "cutting women down to size."

Within feminist scholarship, it is difficult to view the woman who has cos- metic surgery as an agent who—at least to some extent—actively and knowl- edgeably gives shape to her life, albeit under circumstances that are not of her own making. Whether blinded by consumer capitalism, oppressed by patriar- chal ideologies, or inscribed within the discourses of femininity, the woman who opts for the "surgical fix" marches to the beat of a hegemonic system— a system that polices, constrains, and inferiorizes her. If she plays the beauty game, she can only do so as a "cultural dope" (Garfinkel 1967)—as a duped victim of false consciousness or as a normalized object of disciplinary regimes.

While I share this critical assessment of the feminine beauty system and the cultural discourses and practices that inferiorize the female body, it is my con- tention that it is only part of the story. Moreover, in the case of cosmetic surgery, it is a story that may miss the point altogether. It is my contention that considerably more than beauty is at stake when women place their bodies under the surgeon's knife. Understanding why women have cosmetic surgery requires taking a closer look at how women themselves make sense of their decisions in the light of their embodied experiences before and after surgery.

This chapter is based on my research on women's narratives about cosmetic surgery (Davis 1995). Here I begin with the reasons women provide for having their appearance altered surgically. This is followed by an exploration of the process a woman goes through when she has cosmetic surgery. Then, based on an in-depth analysis of one women's narrative, I show how far reaching this transformation is. Cosmetic surgery transforms more than a woman's appearance; it transforms her identity as well. In conclusion, I discuss what a narrative approach to cosmetic surgery means for feminist scholarship on women's involvement in the beauty system.

SURGICAL STORIES

My inquiry spanned a period of several years. I conducted narrative interviews (e.g., Gergen and Gergen 1988 and 1993; Sarbin 1986; Shotter and Gergen 1989; Stanley 1990) with women who had already had, or were planning to have, some kind of cosmetic surgery. In some cases, I was able to talk to women both before and after their operations. The interviews were conducted in my home, or the woman's home, and later in a clinical setting.

I spoke with women who had undergone many kinds of surgery: from a relatively simple ear correction or a breast augmentation to—in the most extreme case—having the whole face reconstructed. My interest being in surgery "for looks," I did not talk to women who had reconstructive surgery as a result of trauma, illness, or a congenital birth defect.

Since the research was conducted in the Netherlands, where cosmetic surgery was—until recently—included in the national health care package, the recipients came from a variety of socioeconomic backgrounds. Some were professional women or academics, others were cashiers or domestic workers, and some were full-time housewives and mothers. Some were married, some single, some heterosexual, some lesbian. Some were feminists; others were not. They ranged in age from a seventeen-year-old schoolgirl whose mother took her in for a breast augmentation (a bit like the ritual of buying the first bra) to a successful, middle-aged business woman seeking a face-lift in order to "fit into the corporate culture."

These women told me about their history of suffering because of their appearance, how they decided to have their bodies altered surgically, their experiences with the operation itself, and their assessments of the outcome of the surgery. While their stories involved highly varied experiences of embodiment as well as different routes toward deciding to have cosmetic surgery, the act of having their bodies altered surgically invariably constituted a biographical "turning point" (Denzin 1989)—a point from which they could look backward at the past to make sense of their decision and forward to the future in order to anticipate what it would mean for them. Their stories were organized in such a way that cosmetic surgery became viewable as an understandable and, indeed, unavoidable course of action in the light of their particular biographical circumstances.

BEING ORDINARY

None of the women I spoke with had cosmetic surgery for the reasons many of us think they do—that is, having their bodies altered so that they could become more beautiful. Indeed, most displayed a noted reluctance to connect their particular problem to beauty and even went to great lengths to assure me that it had nothing to do with a desire to be more beautiful. This point was driven home in different ways.

Some women assured me that they were not particularly interested in how they looked. "It was never *my* ambition to be Miss World" or "*I* don't have to be some sex bomb" were frequently heard remarks. They would make disparaging comments about other women who were preoccupied with physical attractiveness. For example, a woman who had her breasts "lifted" after her second pregnancy explained that she found face-lifts ridiculous because "wrinkles just go along with getting older." A face-lift candidate, on the other hand, expressed disbelief that any woman could even consider having her breasts augmented. "Breasts just don't make that much difference; it's not like your face. That's really important."

Other women acknowledged that beauty did matter to them and that they, too, worried about how they looked ("what woman doesn't?"). They would produce lengthy lists of their own "beauty problems." For example, a women who had a breast augmentation might complain that she had "never liked the wrinkles on her face" or had always been much too thin ("a real bean pole"). A face-lift candidate would sigh that she "would give anything for bigger breasts" or "really hated having such hairy legs." Others admitted that they would love to have different bodies—bigger breasts, fewer wrinkles, slimmer thighs. However, they would "never consider cosmetic surgery for something like that."

For the most part, the women I spoke with insisted that their reasons for having cosmetic surgery were of another order. In their cases, one—and only one—part of their bodies—this nose or these ears, breasts, or hips—was perceived as being too different, too abnormal, too out-of-the-ordinary to be endured. They didn't feel "at home" in their bodies; this particular body part just didn't "*belong*" to the rest of her body or to the person each felt she was. As one woman who had a breast reduction explained: "I know a lot of people think big breasts are sexy, but I'm just not that kind of person. I'm basically a small-breasted type. That's just who I am." In short, women who have cosmetic surgery want to be ordinary. They were not primarily concerned with becoming more beautiful; they just wanted to be "like everyone else."

Ironically, I did not necessarily share these women's conviction that they were physically abnormal or different. Their dissatisfaction had, in fact, little to do with intersubjective standards for acceptable or "normal" feminine appearance. For example, when I spoke with women who were contemplating having cosmetic surgery, I rarely noticed the "offending" body part, let alone understood why it required surgical alteration. From their stories, I could not help but notice that they were generally able to acquire jobs, find partners, produce families, and, in general, lead fairly ordinary lives despite their problems with their appearance. In other words, their appearance and the circumstances of their lives did not seem noticeably different from those of women who do not have cosmetic surgery.

While women's bodily imperfections were often invisible to me, their pain was not. As they told me about the devastating effects their appearance had on their sexuality, their relationships, their feelings about themselves, and their ability to move about in the world, their distress and anguish were utterly convincing. Despite the differences in the specific circumstances that led to a woman's decision to have cosmetic surgery, the experience of suffering was the common feature of their stories. Thus, cosmetic surgery was presented as the only way to alleviate suffering that had passed beyond what any woman should "normally" have to endure. It was an extraordinary solution for an extraordinary problem.

TRANSFORMING THE BODY, TRANSFORMING THE SELF

Cosmetic surgery is not the answer to women's problems with their appearance. A new body does not automatically provide a brand-new self. Contrary to media promises of an exciting new life in the fast lane, the women I spoke with described their lives after surgery as still constrained by the mundane problems and worries that were there prior to the surgery. Nevertheless, they indicated that there had been a transformation. This transformation required a long and often painful process of renegotiating their relationships to their bodies as well as their sense of self.

In order to show just how complex and far reaching this process was, I will now take a look at one narrative in depth. It is the story of a particular woman, whom I shall call Diana. Her narrative—like the narratives of the other women I spoke with—describes what led to the decision to have cosmetic surgery, how she experienced the operation and its outcome, and how she made sense of the events, after the fact. I have selected her case as a particularly good illustration of the transformation involved in the act of having one's appearance altered surgically. There are several reasons for this. To begin with, Diana had the most extreme and extensive operation. Her entire face was reconstructed, requiring several hours under anesthesia, intensive care, a lengthy hospital stay, and a long and painful recovery period. Moreover, her face was the object of an operation that, literally, made her unrecognizable—to her friends, her family, and even herself.[1] A physical transformation of such magnitude not only requires some getting used to, but presumably affects one's sense of who one is in dramatic ways as well. And, finally, Diana was unusually articulate about her motives for having her face altered. She used the interview as an opportunity to reflect on the implications of her experiences for how she felt about her body, her relations with other people, and her sense of self.

DIANA'S STORY

Diana is an attractive schoolteacher in her mid-thirties, married, and the mother of a nine-year-old daughter. Her story begins with the statement that she was a perfectly ordinary-looking child until the age of ten when her teeth suddenly began to protrude. Braces did not help and she became "super ugly"—the object of constant harassment from other children. Throughout her childhood, she suffered from feeling different from everyone else. By the time she reached adolescence, she had found ways to compensate for her appearance, however. She was good at making friends, successful in school, and "knew how to make the most of her looks." Although she remained secretly convinced that she was an outsider—"the perennial wallflower"—she also believed that she had managed to overcome her problems with her appearance. However, this turned out to be just the proverbial "calm before the storm." Diana's conviction that she had finally got her life under control was rudely shattered during her first teaching job. Confronted with the usual problems of disciplining a class, she realized that she hadn't escaped her problems with her appearance after all. Her students teased her mercilessly about her face, and she discovered painfully that she was back to square one. She was devastated at the realization that she was still trapped by how she looked. What she had known all along was confirmed: her body would determine how her life would be. Unable to escape its constraints, she was doomed to a life of misery.

The turning point in Diana's story was a conversation with a friend who had had cosmetic dentistry done on her teeth. After much deliberation, Diana decided to make an appointment with a plastic surgeon. She described her astonishment at seeing photographs of people who had had cosmetic surgery done on their faces. For the first time, she realized that she was not so different, after all. She was no longer the exception, but one among many others. Paradoxically, cosmetic surgery almost seemed like the "normal" thing to do.

The operation itself was a terrible ordeal, and she had to admit that the outcome had been disappointing at first. She did not look nearly as good as she had expected. Nevertheless, she had no regrets about having taken the step. Her primary feeling was relief. As she explained, no one made comments about her looks any more. She had become unnoticeable, invisible. "That's the main thing. I've got a nice face now. I'm just ordinary."

Trajectories of Suffering

Diana's initial narrative took the form of a trajectory. This concept has been used by social scientists to describe the process of suffering that people with bodily disorders go through as they lose control over their bodies and then, through their bodies, over their lives (Strauss and Glaser 1970; Riemann and Schütze 1991). In a narrative about cosmetic surgery, the trajectory begins with the recipient's realization that something is seriously amiss with her body. Gradually, she comes to see her body as different, as uprooted from the mundane world and its normal course of affairs (Riemann and Schütze 1991, 345). As she discovers that she can't do anything to alleviate the problem, she is overcome by hopelessness, despair, and, finally, resignation. Her body becomes a prison from which there is no escape.

In this context, cosmetic surgery becomes a way to "interrupt" the trajectory. By having her face remade, the would-be recipient can obtain—like Diana—an acceptable appearance ("just a nice face"). More important, however, cosmetic surgery allows her to extricate herself from what has become a downward spiral. It is no wonder, then, that women who have cosmetic surgery describe their experiences with exhilaration or even triumph. As Diana put it, "It gave me a kick, like, I'll be damned, but *I really did it.*"

Interrupting the trajectory is only the beginning, however. Cosmetic surgery stories tend to be recycled—that is, told and retold, sometimes as many as five times in a single interview. Just as the narrator has brought her tale to a triumphant end and has announced that she has told "everything there is to tell," she will often pick up her story once again.

Let us take a look at another, and somewhat different, rendition of Diana's experience with cosmetic surgery.

Biographical Work

Diana spent more than half of the interview going back over her initial narrative and unraveling the implications of the operation for her feelings about her body, her sense of self, and her relationships. It turned out that the operation had not provided a panacea for her problems with her appearance, but had generated some new problems as well.

"Having your whole face re-done is not like having a breast reduction where no one notices afterwards that you've had anything done." Diana described going back to work and feeling as though she were "on stage." Her students and colleagues kept glancing at her, obviously unsure whether she was the same teacher they had had before the summer break. While most people eventually recognized her by her voice and movements, others walked right past her. She recalled her shock when one of her colleagues entered the staff room at school and looked straight at her, inquiring "Do you know where I can find Diana?" The biggest problem, however, was that she had difficulties seeing her face as her own. She recalled looking in the mirror or seeing herself in photographs and thinking: "This just isn't *me*."

The transformation in Diana's appearance had unpleasant repercussions in her relationships as well. Her parents and brothers and sisters were disapproving. They complained that she had gone out and got rid of what they considered to be "the family face." Rather than supporting her, they were irritated by or critical of her actions. To her dismay, she found that she had become an outsider, and she had to rethink her own position within her family.

And, finally, Diana had to make sense of her "new" appearance in terms of her biography. A good example of how she managed this occurred toward the end of the interview. After explaining how she had come to terms with the reactions of friends and family and could now accept her face, she asked me whether I would like to see some photographs. Opening an old album, she proceeded to show me snapshots of herself that were taken before the operation—as a little girl swinging in her backyard, playing with girlfriends, or posing with the family at a birthday party. "See—there I am—I was the cute, petted, youngest child who everyone adored," she explained. She then showed me pictures of herself as a teenager—"all arms and legs and with those *terrible* teeth." Suddenly, she looked up and with a big grin and announced that it was "almost as though I am back to the way I was before, back to the beginning. *That* face fit me much better than the one I got later."

Thus, Diana's narrative reduces the history of suffering that was so central to her initial story to little more than an interlude. Cosmetic surgery is now presented as more than a means to interrupt a trajectory of suffering; it has, more generally, restored continuity to her biography.

Cosmetic surgery is an event that divides a woman's life into a before and an after.[2] This necessitates some biographical reconstruction. Women's life histories before surgery need to be integrated with their accounts of their lives after it. This reconstruction process entails going back over the initial narrative and engaging in "biographical work"—that is, the activity of recalling, rehearsing, interpreting, and redefining, which accompanies any event that disturbs, disorders, or simply alters a person's biography (Riemann and Schütze 1991, 339).

While such biographical reconstructions were an essential ingredient of women's surgical stories, they proved insufficient for making sense of the transformation they experienced. Cosmetic surgery is a dramatic and unsettling action. It therefore requires justification.

Let me return again to Diana.

Justifications and Explanations

As we have seen, much of Diana's story was focused on the importance of cosmetic surgery as a means for ending her suffering and reconstructing her biography. She took the perspective of a protagonist who had a long history of feeling different because of her appearance. Cosmetic surgery was defended as a way to become ordinary or "just a nice face." However, in other parts of her narrative, Diana took a different stance altogether.

She explained, for example, that she did not find appearance particularly important after all. It was only relevant in a very "superficial" way, but had never made any "real" difference where her friends were concerned. Or, she recalled how people had warned her that the operation might made her a completely different person, but that this was clearly "ridiculous." She insisted that in *her* experience the only thing that had "really" changed was her looks. Or, she went back to the problem of harassment and described her sympathy for the "irritation" that "you naturally feel toward people who are deviant in some way." After all, she felt the same; *she* didn't like the way she had looked before the operation either. Moreover, she had discovered that she could be just as critical as the next person, when all was said and done. "It's harmless, you know. That's just the way people are."

In addition to minimizing the centrality of appearance in her own life, Diana presented herself as someone with "the usual beauty problems." "Hairy legs—now *that's* a problem, let me tell you." She laughingly regaled me with stories about the indignities of having legs waxed or brave attempts to "just let it grow." Having become an ordinary-looking person herself, she became more critical of the practice of cosmetic surgery. For example, she announced that she would "love to have bigger breasts or a different nose" but "where do you draw the line?" There has to be a limit to "all that manipulation of your body. . . . it's not like just taking an aspirin or something."

By relativizing an action that would otherwise set her apart from other women who are neither as dissatisfied with their appearance as she had been nor so willing to take such drastic measures to alter it, Diana puts the finishing touch on her transformation. She tells how she had, at long last, reentered the fold and become "just like everyone else."

Justifications, like trajectories and biographical work, are an ongoing feature of women's narratives about cosmetic surgery. Narratives are interspersed with argumentative sequences whereby they will often defend their actions one moment, explaining that cosmetic surgery had been necessary in their particular case, only to do an about-face and distance themselves from the practice. It is almost as if an audience of critics is lurking on the sidelines, just waiting to attack. While these reversals seem at first glance to be contradictory, a closer look at their arguments reveals that they are part and parcel of these women's attempts to come to terms with their transformation.

It is not unusual for individuals to arrange debates with themselves, both "internally" or in conversations, whereby they advocate a particular position one moment, only to take the other side in the next. This may, indeed, be what thinking is all about—the way we make sense of ourselves and the world around us (Billig 1987 and 1991; Billig et al. 1988). Thus, by both advocating cosmetic surgery and also "taking the other side," women can work through their own ambivalences about an action that is neither self-explanatory nor unproblematic for them. More generally, their justifications display what makes cosmetic surgery both desirable and problematic, necessary and optional, constraint and choice—all in one.

In conclusion, the in-depth analysis of Diana's story shows that cosmetic surgery entails more than the alteration of a woman's appearance. It also involves the ongoing transformation of her sense of self. Cosmetic surgery is, therefore, an intervention in identity.

NEGOTIATING IDENTITY

Identity is a contested concept. Most prosaically, it refers to a person's sense of self. However, by identity, I am not referring to the empiricist self of social psychology—that is, that unified core of stable traits that is thought to reside in each individual. Nor do I believe in the autonomous (disembodied and disembedded) self of Enlightenment philosophy. On the contrary, I am treating identity here as a process by which an individual discursively constructs a sense of self. Identity entails the ongoing integration of possible perspectives and versions of who an individual is into a coherent and meaning-ful life history. These possible versions are not idiosyncratic or individual, but part of a cultural web of narratives available to the individual (e.g., Benhabib 1992).

Narratives about cosmetic surgery reveal how the surgical transformation of the body both constrains and enables a woman to renegotiate her identity. Just how complex the process of negotiating identity can be is illustrated in the way women tell and retell their stories about cosmetic surgery.

Women's initial narratives present their bodies as ugly, abhorrent, or deviant and their sense of self as irrevocably disordered. Their experience of embodi-ment is organized as a trajectory—a vicious circle or downward spiral. Cos-metic surgery emerges as an imminently plausible and, indeed, necessary course of action. This story of self is about *being different:* "correcting," which is the raison d'être of cosmetic surgery.

In retelling the story, women take a meta-stance, reflecting on what the transformation of their bodies means for who they were before the operation and who they have become after it. Their narratives weave past and present together, thereby integrating their "new" bodies into their life histories. This story of self is about *continuity:* the creation of a coherent biography.

In explaining their reasons and doubts about the surgery, they undertake yet another reconstruction. This time, however, the vantage point of critical dis-tance is adopted. Women deconstruct their initial narratives by showing that, when all is said and done, they are no different from anyone else. This story of self is about returning to *life as usual:* the normalizing of the transformation.

Thus, cosmetic surgery does not only represent the constraints and limita-tions of femininity. It allows some women to renegotiate their relationship to their bodies, and through their bodies, to themselves. In other words, it opens up possibilities for biographical reconstruction and opportunities for women to redefine their sense of self.

In the final part of this chapter, I return to the feminist critique of the fem-inine beauty system and the tendency to view women who have cosmetic sur-gery as the "cultural dopes" of that system. What are the broader implications of a biographical approach for understanding women's involvement in cos-metic surgery, and what does this mean for feminist scholarship on beauty, femininity, and the female body?

EMBODIED SUBJECTS?

Cosmetic surgery is a cultural product of late modernity. It can only emerge as a "solution" to women's problems with their appearance in a culture where the surgical alteration of the body is both readily available and socially acceptable (Bordo 1993). It requires a culture with an unshakable conviction in the technological "fix"—the endless makeability and remakeability of ourselves through our bodies. It requires a culture with a dualistic conception of body and mind, in which surgery enables us to enact our intention upon our bodies. And, last but not least, it requires a culture where gender/power relations are typically enacted in and through women's bodies—that is, a culture in which women must negotiate their identities vis-à-vis their appearance.

In her phenomenology of female body experience, the feminist political theorist Iris Young (1990b) has argued that the "typical" contradiction of feminine embodiment in Western, highly industrialized societies is the tension between the female subject as embodied agent and the female body as object. On the one hand, a woman is the person whose body it is, the subject who enacts her projects and aims through her body. Like men, women experience their bodies as vehicles for enacting their desires or reaching out in the world. On the other hand, women are objectified bodies. In a gendered social order, they are socially defined through their bodies. Under constant critical surveillance by others, women begin to experience their own bodies at a distance. They view themselves as the objects of the intentions and manipulations of others.

Given this tension in women's bodily experience, it is hardly surprising that many women have difficulties feeling at ease, let alone at home, in their bodies. The body is both the site of their entrapment as well as the vehicle for expressing and controlling who they are. Although the objectification of the female body is part and parcel of the situation of most Western women and accounts for a shared sense of bodily alienation, women are also agents—that is, knowledgeable and active subjects who attempt to overcome their alienation, to act upon the world themselves instead of being acted upon by others. They may not be able to "transcend" their bodies as the male subject presumably can,[3] but, as subjects, neither can they ever be entirely satisfied with a rendition of themselves as nothing but a body. Women must, therefore, live a contradiction. As Young (1990b, 144) puts it:

> As human she is a free subject who participates in transcendence, but her situation as a woman denies her that subjectivity and transcendence.

It is in the context of this disempowering tension of feminine embodiment—the objectification of women as "just bodies" and the desire of the female subject to act upon the world—that cosmetic surgery must be located.

In conclusion, cosmetic surgery is not simply the expression of the cultural constraints of femininity, nor is it a straightforward expression of women's oppression or of the normalization of the female body through the beauty system. Cosmetic surgery can enable some women to alleviate unbearable suffering, reappropriate formerly hated bodies, and reenter the mundane world of femininity where beauty problems are routine and—at least to some extent—manageable. It is not a magical solution. Nor does it resolve the problems of feminine embodiment, let alone provide the path to liberation. Cosmetic surgery does, however, allow the individual woman to renegotiate her relationship to her body and, in so doing, construct a different sense of self. In a gendered social order where women's possibilities for action are limited, and more often than not ambivalent, cosmetic surgery can, paradoxically, provide an avenue toward becoming an embodied subject rather than remaining an objectified body.

NOTES

I would like to thank Willem de Haan, Hans-Jan Kuipers, and Helma Lutz for their helpful comments.

1. Faces are particularly powerful cultural symbols of identity. The face is alternatively regarded as representing who a person really is ("everyone has the face she deserves") or distorting or disguising a person's true character. This mirror/mask dichotomy belongs to Western notions about the relationship between the face and the self (Strauss 1969; Synnott 1990).

2. This is the shared cultural format for cosmetic surgery narratives. It can be found in many contexts: for example, women's narratives, in the slide show accompanying a surgeon's lecture, or in the popular press with its stories of surgical successes and failures, or—more implicitly—in women's more routine beauty practices (e.g., Smith 1990, who shows how advertisements for makeup "work" by requiring women to indexically imagine their present bodies before and how they would look following the application of eyeliner).

3. Obviously, men never fully transcend their bodies. The notion of the disembodied masculine subject—the mind without a body—is, like the objectified female body—the body without a mind—a fiction and has been amply criticized in feminist theory (e.g., Bordo 1986; Code 1991).

5

Surgical Passing: Why Michael Jackson's Nose Makes "Us" Uneasy

Several months ago, I had a conversation with some of my feminist colleagues about women's involvement in cosmetic surgery. Everyone agreed that cosmetic surgery to meet the ideals of *feminine* beauty is oppressive. Nevertheless, they conceded, an individual woman might benefit from having her body altered surgically and should, therefore, be allowed that choice. They did not believe in a blanket rejection of cosmetic surgery, but rather in taking a nuanced, critical stance: cosmetic surgery is acceptable in individual cases but should be treated in general with caution.

I then brought up the use of cosmetic surgery to eradicate signs of *ethnicity*. As an example, I mentioned the increasing numbers of Asian women undergoing double eyelid surgery to make their eyes look wider and, presumably, more "Western" (Kaw 1993). My colleagues were incensed. They insisted that this was completely reprehensible. When I tried to pin them down about what it was that made surgery for altering "racial" or ethnic features different than a breast augmentation for enhancing femininity, they looked uncomfortable. They hesitated and finally admitted that they didn't know. "It just feels different, somehow worse."

This discussion left me with several questions. I was struck by the immediacy and intensity of my colleagues' response that cosmetic surgery on "racial" or ethnic features was not only different, but also decidedly worse (politically and ethically) than a breast augmentation or a face-lift. My initial inclination was to view this reaction as an expression of the anger, uneasiness, or—for the white women among us—guilt, which the racism inherent in such surgery is likely to evoke. At the same time, however, I was somewhat uneasy about their relative lack of concern when it came to cosmetic surgery for enhancing femininity. Isn't any recipient of cosmetic surgery, regardless of gender, ethnicity or nationality, sexual orientation or age, engaged in negotiating her identity in contexts where differences in embodiment can evoke unbearable suffering?

It is, of course, possible that the shocked response of my colleagues to the surgical "Westernization" of Asian women's eyelids was a reflection of the relative lack of attention given to the practice in public discourse about cosmetic surgery. Women have always been the primary recipients of all kinds of cosmetic surgery (including surgery for ethnic features). Feminists have tended to link the cultivation of the body in the name of beauty to femininity. Given the ubiquity of viewing cosmetic surgery through the lens of gender, surgical interventions for enhancing femininity may seem so ordinary that they have become—more or less—acceptable, while surgery for eradicating ethnic features can still be counted on to elicit surprise and disapproval.

But perhaps the explanation lay elsewhere. I began to wonder whether our discussion might not be another rendition of the old and familiar debate about hierarchies of oppression. It reminded me of countless discussions I have had in the past with feminists who argue that gender (not class or race) is the primary category of difference and with antiracists who maintain, just as decisively, that racism, not sexism, is the enemy most deserving of our critical attention. This kind of dualistic thinking has been convincingly debunked by Floya Anthias and Nira Yuval-Davis (1992), Avtar Brah (1996), Naomi Zack (1997), Valerie Smith (1998), Jacquelyn Zita (1998), and many others, who have argued that gender and race are not separate systems of domination, but rather intersecting and mutually constitutive features of any social practice or historical context. This view—and it is one that I share—suggests that the task facing feminists today is not deciding whether gender or race is more relevant, but rather how these and other categories of difference intersect to produce specific constellations of hierarchy, exclusion, or exploitation.

In this chapter, I will attempt to make sense of the unease evoked by "ethnic cosmetic surgery"[1] and the issues that it raises for feminists and other critical scholars. Taking a brief look at its history and its current manifestations, I will situate the practice in the legacy of "racial science" and contemporary debates about the politics of beauty. The case of Michael Jackson—arguably the most well-known recipient of this kind of cosmetic surgery—will provide the case in point for discussing two separate but related questions. The first concerns how cosmetic surgery for eradicating signs of "ethnicity" might be different than cosmetic surgery for enhancing femininity, and the second concerns whether ethnic cosmetic surgery has more serious normative or political implications than other forms of cosmetic surgery.

ETHNIC COSMETIC SURGERY: A HISTORICAL SKETCH

As practice, ethnic cosmetic surgery is not new. Since the emergence of cosmetic surgery at the turn of the twentieth century, individuals in the United States and Europe have not only looked to cosmetic surgery as a way to enhance their appearance. It has also enabled them to minimize or eradicate physical signs that they believe mark them as "Other"—"Other" invariably meaning other than the dominant or more desirable racial or ethnic group (Haiken 1997, 175–76).

In central Europe throughout the nineteenth century, the "Other" was the Jew. Stereotypical images proliferated, marking the Jewish body as different, deformed, and pathological. Jews were thought to have flat feet (making them unfit for military duty), disgusting skin diseases (*Judenkratze*), elongated ears with fleshy earlobes ("Moritz ears"), characteristic noses ("nostrility"), and, of course, genitalia "damaged" by circumcision (Gilman 1991). These racial markers were associated with social stigmas of weakness, illness, and degeneracy, thereby making appearance an obstacle for the assimilation of Jews into Aryan society. Early cosmetic surgeons like Jacques Josef, the founder of modern rhinoplasty and himself an "acculturated German Jew," developed surgical procedures that allowed Jewish patients to become "ethnically invisible."[2]

In the United States, cosmetic surgery became popular in the wake of large-scale immigration at the turn of the twentieth century. The first nose correction was performed by John Roe for the "pug nose"—a feature that was associated with Irish immigrants[3] and negative qualities of character like slovenliness and doglike servility (hence the term "pug"). Nose surgery was later performed on European immigrants (Jews, Italians, and others of Mediterranean or eastern European descent) as well as on white Americans who were anxious that they "looked Jewish" (Haiken 1997). Following World War II, cosmetic surgery became popular among Koreans, Chinese, Japanese, and Asian Americans to create folded eyelids ("Western eyes"). More recently, African Americans have begun to alter their noses and lips through cosmetic surgery.[4] By 1998, it was estimated that of the 2.8 million cosmetic surgery procedures performed in the United States, 19.6 percent of the procedures were performed on patients who were not Caucasian—that is, of Asian, Hispanic, Native American, or African American descent (Matory 1998, xix).

Ethnic cosmetic surgery is typically oriented to the most identifiable and caricatured facial features—for Jews, noses; for Asians, eyes and noses; and for African Americans, noses and lips. However, no body part is safe from being racially marked. For example, in Rio de Janeiro, "pendulous breasts" are linked to the lower classes, which are imagined as black—an image that has its roots in the institution of black slavery that was not abolished in Brazil until 1888 (Gilman 1999, 225).

The emergence of ethnic cosmetic surgery cannot be separated from scientific ideas about race, which permeated the popular imagination throughout the nineteenth century. Western science has historically played a dubious role in legitimating social inequalities based on both sex and race.[5] However, scientific discourse on race intensified and was institutionalized as "racial science" during the second half of the nineteenth century, providing a "series of lenses through which human variation was constructed, understood, and experienced" (Stepan and Gilman 1993). The doctrine of the Great Chain of Being constructed racial groups as discrete and immutable entities arranged hierarchically along a continuum with God and the white European on the top and the African and orangutan at the bottom. In this way, social inequalities stemming from rampant slave trade and colonial expansion could be justified as the inevitable consequences of "natural hierarchies" (Gould 1981; Stepan 1982; Harding 1993). Biologists and physical anthropologists developed complex racial taxonomies based on phenotypical attributes like the shape and size of the skull (for men) or pelvis (for women), the form of the nose or mouth, skin color, and hair texture.[6] These anatomical features were typically mixed with descriptions of character. For example, the Irish—at that time considered a race—were thought to be directly descended from the big-eared Cro-Magnon man, and the face of "Bridget McBruiser" with her low forehead, shifty eyes, and slovenly demeanor was frequently contrasted in physiognomy books with Florence Nightingale's "English" beauty and obvious moral worth (Gilman 1999, 94; see, also, Stepan 1982).

If white northern European features constituted the standard against which all other "races" were measured, it was hardly surprising that individuals with features that marked them as "Other" than white or northern European would want to hide visible clues that they saw as having unfavorable or stigmatic connotations (Haiken 1997, 186).

For immigrants and members of marginalized groups, the newly emerging medical specialty of cosmetic surgery seemed to provide the solution. It offered a way to achieve upward mobility and assimilation in a culture that defined certain people as different and, more importantly, inferior, by virtue of their appearance. According to Haiken, cosmetic surgery allows individuals to become "ethnically anonymous."

Gilman takes this argument one step further, referring to cosmetic surgery as a form of "passing." Passing refers to an individual assuming a new identity in order to escape the subordination and oppression accompanying one identity and access the privileges and status of another (Ginsberg 1996, 3).

While it can refer to homosexuals passing as heterosexuals or women passing as men, passing is most commonly associated with discourses of racial difference and the legacy of slavery. In the United States, where the color line was rigidly enforced through the "one-drop rule" and miscegenation laws, many light-skinned blacks left their families and communities and took on a white identity.

Although Gilman situates his discussion in postwar Germany where Jewish individuals wanted to pass as non-Jews and German patients wanted to be "cured" of possessing a "too Jewish" physiognomy, he regards surgical passing as a much broader phenomenon.

In his view, the desire to eliminate difference and belong to a more desirable group is not limited to those with ethnically marked features. Passing is the basic motivation for any form of cosmetic surgery, whether ethnically marked features are involved or not. Thus, face-lifts make it possible for the middle-aged to "pass" as youthful, and breast augmentations help flat-chested women to "pass" as sexy. In short, cosmetic surgery is a form of "surgical passing."

SURGICAL DISCOURSE: FROM "RACE" TO "INDIVIDUAL ENHANCEMENT"

While medical historians like Gilman and Haiken have explicitly linked the emergence of cosmetic surgery to "race" and the practice of passing, contemporary medical texts seem reluctant to tackle the "race issue." Most surgeons treat cosmetic surgery as a beauty issue. They explain their patients' desire to have their bodies altered as a consequence of the universal human desire for a pleasing and attractive appearance. In a culture where self-improvement is almost a moral imperative, it is apparently only "natural" and "normal" for anyone—particularly if she is a woman—to want to look her best.[7]

In 1998, a coffee-table-sized, 412-page textbook with glossy pages and numerous color photographs appeared with the title *Ethnic Considerations in Facial Aesthetic Surgery*. Twenty-nine contributors—all reputable cosmetic surgeons—addressed psychological, anatomical, and cultural considerations in cosmetic facial surgery for African American, Asian, Hispanic, Middle-Eastern, Filipino-Polynesian, and—to a considerably lesser degree—northern European patients.

Such a textbook was necessary for various reasons. According to the editor, W. Earle Matory Jr., himself a pioneer in the field, the development of cosmetic surgery has up until now been influenced by northern European beauty ideals. This has become increasingly problematic, given the fact that

35 percent of the U.S. population today is not Caucasian. Procedures are, therefore, required that take their special needs into account. In his view, ethnic cosmetic surgery is simply a matter of going with the flow—of adapting the available technology to encompass a growing group of potential patients. Other authors situate cosmetic surgery for the "ethnic patient" in the changing political climate. According to this line of reasoning, cosmetic surgery is a newly won "right" for previously excluded groups. Just as people of color should have access to higher education, well-paid jobs, and homes in suburbia, they should be able to take advantage of cosmetic surgery.

All authors emphasize, however, that cosmetic surgery on "ethnic features" is not about eradicating ethnicity. The goal is rather to create the ideal characteristics of beauty within each ethnic category (Matory 1998, xix). Patients who "reject" their ethnic background make poor candidates for cosmetic surgery. The suitable patient for ethnic cosmetic surgery is, in contrast, the individual with a "pragmatic desire to improve appearance" (Gorney 1998, 5).

Despite this insistence that each ethnicity has its own beauty, the authors are very concerned about finding a "universal standard of beauty" by which their interventions on the "ethnic patient" can be justified. To this end, they draw upon anthropometric measures like the Frankfurter horizontal, the neoclassical canons of facial proportion, and the golden aesthetic of facial relationships as neutral, nonethnic standards of beauty. Of course, this standard is none other than the classical Greek model. The faces of men and women from different ethnic groups are analyzed against this model, and features that do not match are established as objects for surgical intervention.

Although this ideal standard of beauty is clearly necessary for developing and justifying procedures for changing "ethnic" features, surgeons rigorously—and repeatedly—deny that the ideal has any connection with whiteness or Western ethnicities. The result is the best of both worlds: a model that brings the "accepted standard of beauty" to an appearance that "retains its ethnic character" (Rohrich and Kenkel 1998, 96).

THE POLITICS OF BEAUTY

Norms of appearance that define certain groups as less attractive invariably raise normative questions. They cannot be viewed as simply a matter of "whimsical aesthetic preference" or the individual's "right" to look better, but rather draw upon a broader system of attitudes and actions in which particular categories of individuals—women or people of color—are devalued, while men and whites are privileged (Little 1998). In societies plagued by social inequalities, cosmetic surgery in the cases of disadvantaged groups involves injustice and is, therefore, a matter of politics rather than aesthetics.

Feminists have a long tradition of situating beauty ideals and women's involvement in beauty practices in a political context (Wolf 1991; Bordo 1993; Davis, 1991 and 1995). They argue that beauty is integral to the construction of femininity in a gendered social order. The female sex is idealized as the incarnation of beauty, while the bodies of most ordinary women tend to be treated as inferior and in constant need of improvement. Cosmetic surgery is regarded as a particularly insidious way to discipline the female body—to literally, "cut women down to size." Feminists have been fairly unanimous in their rejection of cosmetic surgery as dangerous and demeaning for women. While they are reluctant to blame individual women who look to cosmetic surgery as a solution to their suffering, feminists have tended to view such women as the duped and manipulated victims of the feminine beauty culture. Since cosmetic surgery is—almost by definition—"bad news" for women, it is difficult to attribute agency or "choice" to women's desire for surgical "enhancement."

Racialized standards of beauty have provoked similar controversies. The Black Power movement of the sixties made appearance a political issue with the well-known motto "Black is beautiful." Racist (and classist) norms of appearance that equate feminine beauty with long flowing hair, light skin, and aquiline features were criticized as part of a "color caste system" that historically defines black women with kinky hair and African features as "ugly" or undesirable (hooks 1994; Russell, Wilson, and Hall 1992; Mama 1995). The detrimental effects of this devaluation have been considerable, ranging from overt discrimination in the workplace and educational system to pervasive self-hate among people of color. In particular, the popularity of controversial practices like skin bleaching and hair straightening has been the subject of critical attention among critical (feminist) scholars (hooks 1990, 1992, and 1994; Mercer 1994; Rooks 1996; Banks 2000).[8]

While some critics, like bell hooks (1994), situate the desire for light skin and long straight hair unambiguously in the context of "racist imagination" and "colonized black mind set" (179), others take a more nuanced stance. Noliwe Rooks (1996), for example, traces the history of hair straightening, showing how it draws upon discourses of "racial uplift" as well as "self-hate" within the black community and has generated women's communities and possibilities for upward mobility as well as discourses of racial inferiority.

In her study of cosmetic surgery, Eugenia Kaw (1993 and 1994) shows how corrective eyelid surgery among Asian American women goes hand in hand with racialized standards of appearance. In her view, such surgery is "of a different quality" than face-lifts or liposuctions for Anglo-Americans. The desire to create more "open" eyes or "sharpen" noses is a product of racial ideologies that associate Asian features with negative behavioral or intellectual characteristics like dullness, passivity, or lack of emotion (the proverbial

Oriental bookworm). Although all of Kaw's respondents explained that they were "proud to be Asian American" and that they did not want to "look white," she cannot help but notice that the beauty standard they admire includes large eyes with a double eyelid and a more prominent nose—in short, a Caucasian face.

> If the types of cosmetic surgery Asian Americans opt for are truly individual choices, one would expect to see a number of Asians who admire and desire eyes without a crease or a nose without a bridge. (Kaw 1993, 86)

When an Asian American woman explains that she is having double-eyelid surgery because "big eyes look more alert" or because she wants to "optimize her position in the business world" or, simply because she wants to use eye makeup ("just like other women"), Kaw does not take her words at face value. For Asian Americans, the desire for cosmetic surgery is automatically assumed to be "racially" motivated; that is, they are trying to disguise their ethnicity and look more "Western."

> Because the features (eyes and nose) Asian Americans are most concerned about are conventional markers of their racial identity, a rejection of these markers entails, in some sense, a devaluation of not only oneself but also other Asian Americans. It requires having to imitate, if not admire, the characteristics of another group more culturally dominant than one's own (i.e., Anglo Americans) in order that one can at least try to distinguish oneself from one's group. (Kaw 1994, 254)

Thus, cosmetic surgery when undertaken by people of color or the ethnically marginalized is framed in a political discourse of race rather than beauty. Whether they are positioned in a narrative of racial passing or cultural assimilation, ethnic or "racial" minorities generally have less discursive space than their white counterparts for justifying their decisions to have cosmetic surgery. Even when the recipients of such surgery claim—as they often do—that they just want to look better or are simply exercising their right to self-improvement or that they are responding to limitations, which identifiably ethnic features impose on their lives and careers, they tend to be seen as the victims of racist norms (Haiken 1997, 213). By altering their racially marked features, they also run the risk of being accused of denying their racial or ethnic heritage and, in so doing, of undermining or devaluing their "own" ethnic or racial group in its attempts to develop an empowering, non-Caucasian aesthetic. In short, they become "race traitors" (Haiken 1997, 189).

Nowhere is the tendency to "racialize" cosmetic surgery more evident than in the case of its most celebrated recipient, Michael Jackson. His surgical exploits force both whites and people of color to deal with the "race issue" head on and, more generally, to confront one of the most painful and pervasive problems in contemporary U.S. society (Haiken 1997, 177). For this reason, he provides a useful starting point for exploring the unease that ethnic cosmetic surgery evokes.

MICHAEL JACKSON AND THE "RACE ISSUE"

Michael Jackson, the self-designated "King of Pop," is one of the most popular entertainers in the history of American music. From his auspicious beginnings as child singer and dancer in the Jackson 5, he went on to become one of the most prolific and talented performers and songwriters in the eighties and nineties. His album *Thriller* (1982) was the second best-selling record of all time. Jackson's importance for the music world is undisputed, but it is his bizarre behavior that receives the most attention in the media. This includes his wearing tight, flashy clothing and more mascara and eyeliner than most leading ladies; adopting strange disguises like dark glasses and surgical masks; sleeping in a sealed glass, coffinlike shell, originally developed for burn victims, in order to stay young; and—last but not least—undergoing multiple cosmetic surgeries.

Jackson has had at least four rhinoplasties as well as numerous "fine-tuning" operations. The result is a fragile, pointed nose, whittled away to almost nothing, that gives his face a skeletal look. His nose is a running joke among plastic surgeons on both sides of the Atlantic ("Thank God, I'm not that guy's surgeon"). Jackson has also had a cleft put in his chin, cheek implants, his lower lip "thinned," and probably some face-lifting. Judging by the ghostlike pallor of his face, he has made ample use of skin bleaching agents and heavy white pancake makeup. The Michael Jackson of today bears no resemblance to the cute, dark-skinned child of the seventies, with African features, dressed in flower-power pants and sporting a huge Afro.

What does Michael Jackson himself have to say about his dramatic metamorphosis? In his biography, he has claimed that his "only" interest is to "look better." It's a matter of choice: "I can afford it, I want it, so I'm going to have it," he says (Taraborrelli 1991, 420). In this sense, he is no different than countless other well-known celebrity cosmetic surgery junkies like Cher, Dolly Parton, or Pamela Anderson. Jackson clearly uses his identity transformations as a celebrity stunt and integrates them in his music, videos, and private life (see Yuan 1996). As he puts it, the bottom line is that his audience doesn't know who he is and will keep searching until they find out. "And the longer it takes to discover this, the more famous I will be" (Taraborrelli 1991, 388). Thus,

Jackson's surgeries could be treated as a matter of show business utility—of using his body as a vehicle for selling his music.

Critics have not been convinced that Jackson is simply engaging in a celebrity stunt when he has his face altered surgically. However, when asked whether he is trying to become white, Jackson's responses have been typically mercurial. He claims that he is proud to be black, and in a televised conversation with Oprah Winfrey in 1993, he even referred to himself as a "slave to rhythm." Moreover, he insists that he has a skin disorder (vitiligo) and is only using white makeup to cover up his skin depigmentation. Critics have been skeptical, arguing that he could have darkened his white blotches as most patients do. But Jackson can hardly be charged with trying to "pass" as white. He does not seem to be abandoning his origins, as the history of his facial transformations is available to anyone with access to Internet. Perhaps the most accurate reading of how Jackson feels about race is expressed in his song "Black or White": "I am tired of this stuff. . . . I'm not going to spend my life being a color." [9]

Whatever Jackson's "true" sentiments about race are—and I doubt that we will ever know—his new image lends itself to interpretations other than a race change. For example, his surgeries seem to be at least as much about creating a feminine, asexual, or youthful appearance as they are about becoming white. In fact, Jackson has often announced that he would most like to look like Diana Ross. To this end, he has adopted a high, breathy whisper, and rumors have it that he is contemplating a sex change operation. Seen from this angle, Jackson's experiments with androgyny and sexual ambiguity are reminiscent of the playful sexual border crossings of white male icons in popular culture like David Bowie, Mick Jaggar, and Boy George (Mercer 1994, 50). His ethereal, almost deathlike demeanor makes one wonder whether he isn't attempting to transcend the material body altogether, and, in this respect, his surgical antics might best be compared to the surgical performances of the body artist Orlan.[10]

Given the myriad possibilities for understanding Jackson's surgical exploits, it is, therefore, remarkable that the alteration of his racially marked features have, by far, received the most attention in public and scholarly discourse. Michael Awkward (1995) provides a useful map of the debate, which can help clarify if not explain this preoccupation. On the one hand, critics have been concerned about Jackson's motivations and the potential consequences of his cosmetic surgeries. They regard his blanched skin and disfigured African features as a violation of nature, an unnatural act that entails negating his essential identity. Others view Jackson's surgeries as a reflection of racist ideals of appearance, expressing his enslavement to Eurocentric definitions of beauty. His surgeries are a "morbid symptom of a psychologically mutilated black consciousness," representing the pervasive self-hate among blacks that was the object of critique by Black Power advocates (Awkward

1995, 177). On a more strident note, still other critics have argued that Jackson's face is the product of a self-serving desire to achieve fame by becoming white—a "singular infamy in the annals of tomming" (Tate 1992)—nothing less than a "deracializing sell-out."

On the other hand, critics of a more post-structuralist bent have argued that Jackson is better seen as the "exemplary postmodernist actor," who uses the surface of his own body as a text upon which he constantly rearticulates and transforms his image. His surgical feats are not about betrayal of his race, but about transgressing racial boundaries altogether. Despite the historical associations that Jackson's surgeries evoke with racism and passing, they also have a liberatory effect. His face provides a visible assault on any assertion of absolute bodily difference, "crack[ing] open any monolithic notion one might have about the coherent racial self" (Gubar 1997, 249). By transcending the categories of race, Jackson demonstrates in the most embodied way possible that "race" really doesn't matter.

According to Awkward (1995), Jackson's critics can't avoid getting caught up in the debate between race as essence and race as construct. The first group can be criticized for treating "race" as a natural or essentialist category, while the second group pays too little attention to the historical and ideological context that conditions even the most disruptive or utopian racial transgression. While I agree with his conclusion, it does not resolve the issue of why Jackson's bodily transformations remain connected to "race." Whether Jackson is regarded as a "race traitor" or a "race bender," his cosmetic surgeries cannot apparently be seen as anything but racially motivated—as an attempt to deny, efface, or transcend his racial identity. This conviction overrides Jackson's own explanation of his motives. It also predominates over other perfectly plausible interpretations of his actions as, for example, being a "typical" celebrity stunt or an attempt to develop his feminine side or even a valiant attempt to escape the body's materiality altogether.

Michael Jackson confronts his audiences—regardless of their color or political persuasion—with the "race issue" (Haiken 1997). While a white person may be free to experiment with her or his appearance—and this includes indulging in the "surgical fix"—the same experiment takes on a different meaning when undertaken by people of color or the ethnically marginalized.

COSMETIC SURGERY AND
THE ETHICS OF DIFFERENCE

At the outset of this chapter, I raised the question of how ethnic cosmetic surgery is different from other forms of cosmetic surgery and, more specifically, why cosmetic surgery for eliminating signs of "race" or ethnicity seems so much "worse" than cosmetic surgery for a feminine or youthful appearance. A brief foray into cultural and medical perspectives on ethnic cosmetic surgery, both in the past and present, as well as debates about the political implications of such surgery shows that while similar arguments can be made about the surgeries, the discourses in which they are framed are different. Cosmetic surgery for people of color or the ethnically marginalized is about "race," while cosmetic surgery for white Anglos is about beauty.

In *Reshaping the Female Body* (1995), I took issue with the notion that cosmetic surgery is motivated by individuals' desire to be more beautiful. They experience their bodies as different or abnormal and have cosmetic surgery to become ordinary and normal—"just like everyone else." I argued that in a much more profound sense, cosmetic surgery is an intervention in identity rather than an intervention in appearance.

The primary problem with defining cosmetic surgery exclusively in terms of beauty is that recipients are easily cast as frivolous, star struck, or ideologically manipulated.[11] In contrast, by treating cosmetic surgery as an intervention in identity, it becomes easier to take their experiences with their bodies seriously, acknowledge the gravity of their suffering, and understand why—in the face of all its drawbacks—cosmetic surgery might seem like their best course of action under the circumstances.

It seems to me that this perspective should—in principle—be applied to any person who undergoes cosmetic surgery. In other words, *all* recipients of cosmetic surgery should be regarded as negotiating their identities in a context where differences in embodiment can evoke unbearable suffering. While the context that produces such suffering deserves critical attention (and I will be turning to this in a moment), I see no fundamental reason to regard an African American candidate for nose surgery as less "victimized" by cultural beauty ideals or more "traitorous" to his or her community than a white Anglo woman who has her breasts augmented or her face lifted.

While I would argue that cosmetic surgery is best seen as an intervention in identity for everyone regardless of gender or ethnicity, this does not mean that all cosmetic surgeries have the same meaning. Identities are negotiated in specific historical and social contexts in which cultural constructions of race, ethnicity, gender, sexuality, age, and nationality shape how an individual perceives her or his body as well as the kinds of bodily practices that are considered desirable, acceptable, or appropriate for altering the body. Surgical interventions performed on different groups have their own histories of exclusion and inferiorization. The history of the "Jewish nose job," for example, is a different one than the history of eyelid corrections for Asians or lip surgery for African Americans. The alterations that Jacques Josef performed on "assimilated" Jews in the context of European anti-Semitism in the early twentieth century had a different meaning than the ubiquitous nose jobs performed on Jewish teenagers in the early sixties in the United States under the motto: "You had your bat mitzvah, and you got your nose done." In a similar vein, large numbers of affluent young women have their noses "fixed" in Iran every year, declaring that they "just want to look better." Such surgery may well be a class issue, something that young women of a certain social background are entitled to do. However, in the United States when private clinics, catering to the growing community of Iranian exiles, perform the same nose surgery, it falls under the rubric of ethnic cosmetic surgery ("the Middle Eastern nose"). Obviously a contextual understanding of cosmetic surgery would of necessity require unraveling the complicated and contradictory interconnections between different categories of difference (race, ethnicity, class, gender, sexuality, age, able-bodiedness, and more) and their meanings at particular historical periods and specific social locations.

A critique of cosmetic surgery and, more generally, a politics of the body, cannot be reduced to *either* gender *or* race. An exclusive focus on gender would be inadequate for understanding why the practice of cosmetic surgery has been a primarily white, Western enterprise. By the same token, an exclusive focus on race or ethnicity could not account for why most operations on "Jewish noses" or "Oriental eyelids" are performed on women. White women, with their ostensibly "unmarked" identities, participate in the privilege and oppressive mentality of Northern European ideals of a feminine beauty when they have cosmetic surgery, making it a specifically ethnicized and racialized practice as well.

Embodiment involves intersections at the level of the person's experiences with her or his body as well as the cultural meanings attached to the body and body practices. It is precisely these intersections that provide the starting point for a contextualized analysis of cosmetic surgery as cultural phenomenon. In this sense, an analysis of embodiment as well as cosmetic surgery as an intervention in a person's embodied identity belongs squarely within the intersectional frameworks, which I mentioned at the outset of this chapter.

Nowhere is this more apparent than the case of Michael Jackson. His surgical exploits are shaped by, but also transgress, the boundaries of race, gender, age, and sexuality. Jackson's operations demonstrate the spuriousness of categories of race and force his public to see him as an individual in complete control of his bodily image. The image that emerges is a new category, made more captivating and volatile by virtue of its multiple transgressions of masculinity and heterosexuality. At the same time, Jackson's face evokes discomfort. It is a painful reminder of the legacy of slavery and the ubiquitous racism in the United States, which has made and will always make cross-racial "passing" a less-than-playful practice.

A recent image on the Internet speaks louder than words of the inability to disconnect Jackson from this heritage.[12] Appearing in a white satin tuxedo, heavy makeup, and flowing hair, Jackson is shown accepting his trophy from the Rock 'n' Roll Hall of Fame. Juxtaposed to his photograph is a still from the film *Planet of the Apes* (2001), showing one of the leading apes (played by Helena Bonham-Carter) in heavy ape makeup and ape costume, dressed in a shimmering disco suit. The resemblance between the images is unmistakable: their faces and poses are alike, their hair is similar, they are wearing same kind of clothing. Taken alone, the photograph of Jackson is just a record of his moment of fame; the "King of Pop" has "arrived." Together with the photograph of Bonham-Carter, however, the image takes on a different meaning.[13] No matter how far he comes or how great his accomplishments are, Jackson can never escape his (primitive) origins. The Great Chain of Being which placed primates and Africans at the bottom of the hierarchy did not vanish with the "science of race," but apparently continues to shape the popular imagination today.

CONCLUSION

A final word is in order concerning the relative unease that ethnic cosmetic surgery evokes. Cosmetic surgery not only has different meanings depending on the cultural and historical context. It also evokes, as we have seen, different emotional and moral responses. The long history of medicalizing (white) women's bodies as well as the normalization of the female body through the cultural dictates of the feminine beauty system have made cosmetic surgery for white Western women ordinary, routine, and *salonfähig*. The fact that every year millions of women have their breasts augmented or their wrinkles smoothed out is hardly news, let alone a source of discomfort.

In contrast, ethnic cosmetic surgery—at least in some of its forms and in some places—still evokes uneasiness. It is an uncomfortable reminder of the long and disturbing history of slavery, colonialism, and genocide. Jackson's face demonstrates in no uncertain terms that "the tar baby, like the proverbial elephant in the living room, does not vanish just because it is ignored" (Haiken 1997, 227). The "one-drop rule" and the underlying fear of racial mixing is not a relic of the nineteenth century, but lives on in the anxieties of white Americans in the United States today. Any white-skinned person who acknowledges African ancestry, however distant, implicitly acknowledges that he is black—an identity that a white person in the United States might be less than willing to accept given the disentitlement and disempowerment that such an admission could entail. And yet, most Americans who are presently defined as white in the United States have, according to the "one-drop rule," a significant percentage of African ancestry. The fear of exposure and of having to "reinternalize the external scapegoat . . . by which they have sought to escape their own sense of inferiority" (Piper 1996, 256) is perhaps white America's most "shameful" secret.

Ethnic cosmetic surgery evokes ambivalence. As a kind of "surgical passing," it can be viewed as a symptom of "internalized racism" or as a traitorous complicity with oppressive norms of physical appearance. But it cannot be reduced to the straightforward rejection of black or ethnic identity. The sense of unfairness at realizing what is denied to a person because of physical markers like skin color or hair or the shape of a nose may be so overwhelming that a nose job or eyelid correction may feel like an oppositional act—a way to defy the system and get the benefits a person knows she deserves. Adrian Piper (1996) gets it right when she argues that "passing" may not be so much about rejecting blackness (or any other marked identity) as about rejecting an identification with blackness that brings too much pain to be tolerated (244–45).[14]

Ethnic cosmetic surgery is a controversial practice because it touches upon how the construction of race through the body is linked to racist practices of inferiorization and exclusion. It brings up the uncomfortable fact that in ostensibly democratic societies individuals continue to be defined as "Other" and are, therefore, forced to find ways to disguise their "other-ness"—that is, to become invisible—in order to improve their life chances. At a time when wide-scale migrations are, literally, changing the "face" of many European countries and when "race" and racism are the most urgent problems in U.S. society today, "ethnic cosmetic surgery" should make anyone who is even superficially interested in redressing injustice uneasy.

And this is—I believe—as it should be. However, in the face of the enormous expansion of technologies for eradicating differences of all kinds, it is not only our *ability* to feel compassion, concern, or shock that is at stake. Our *inability* to sympathize, our lack of concern, or our numbness toward any individual or group embarking on the "surgical fix" may be equally worthy of our critical attention.

NOTES

For their constructive and helpful comments on various versions of this paper, I would like to thank Cynthia Cockburn, Halleh Gorashi, Barbara Henkes, Lena Inowlocki, Helma Lutz, Sawitri Saharso, Gloria Wekker, Henri Wijsbek, and Dubravka Zarkov. I am deeply grateful to Anna Aalten and Willem de Haan, who have helped me untangle more knots than bear thinking about and who are always willing to take just one more look.

1. I have struggled with the terminology and have not come up with a satisfactory designation. In many medical texts, references to race and ethnicity are oblique ("certain groups are blessed more bountifully in the area of their olfactory organs"). Surgeons avoid the term "race," referring instead to the "ethnic patient" or "ethnic-specific surgery." Historically, "race" has been linked to bodily markers of difference, however spurious, while "ethnicity" tends to be linked to culture. Ethnicity, which is just as constructed as race, is frequently racialized in practice—that is, treated as an embodied characteristic of cultural groups (see, for example, Stepan 1982; Goldberg 1990; Appiah 1996). Since this has also been the case with cosmetic surgery, which—as I will show in this chapter—applies the "science of race" to features that are subsequently classified as "ethnic," I have opted for "ethnic cosmetic surgery."

2. Josef exemplifies the ambiguities of "ethnic cosmetic surgery." His own career was established through his efforts to reshape "Jewish" noses and help individuals "conceal their origins." His own efforts to belong included joining a *Burschenschaft* where he received the obligatory dueling scars as a marker of Aryan manhood. However, Josef could not escape his origins and despite his important contributions to the field would have been forced to resign along with other Jewish physicians when Hitler came into power. It is unclear whether he died of a heart attack or took his own life in 1934, just before he would have been forbidden to practice medicine (Gilman 1991).

3. The Irish were regarded as a "race" in the nineteenth century, while at present they can, at most, lay claim to an "ethnicity"—an interesting fact in the history of the construction of race.

4. The relative underrepresentation of African Americans among cosmetic surgery recipients may be linked to the primacy of skin color as racial marker—a feature that cannot be easily altered through cosmetic surgery. While cosmetic surgery may not be widespread among African Americans, the use of skin-bleaching products is (see Russell, Wilson, and Hall 1992).

5. In the wake of the French Revolution and the ideological call for equality among all, science has been instrumental in generating evidence for "natural" differences between the sexes. Prior to the eighteenth century, thinking about the body was dominated by the "one-sex model"; the woman was understood as man inverted, with the vagina regarded as penis, the vulva as foreskin, the uterus as scrotum, and the ovaries as testicles (Lacqueur 1990). While women were considered inferior to men (they had less heat), it wasn't until the late eighteenth century that women were regarded as having radically different bodies. This shift in thinking—the "two-sex model"—provided a natural basis for the doctrine of separate social spheres, which excluded women from public life and relegated them to a life of domesticity.

6. See Schiebinger (1993) for a good discussion of how sex and race were linked in scientific discourse.

7. In chapter 7, I show that while this trend also applies to men who have cosmetic surgery, a closer look reveals that surgeons do not find men's desire to alter their bodies surgically entirely normal and are, in fact, reluctant to have them as patients.

8. See, also, Carroll 2000 and Taylor 2000 for a discussion of antiracist aesthetics.

9. Michael Jackson, "Black or White," *Dangerous,* Epic Records EK 45400.

10. Orlan and her performances to deconstruct the natural body and the notion of a fixed identity through cosmetic surgery will be discussed in the next chapter.

11. Even feminists are prone to do this. For example, Little (1998) describes the "typical" female cosmetic surgery recipient as a woman who already has a size-eight body but is so distressed by the pictures of super models that she sees in the media that she requests not just one, but a whole series of surgeries: "extensive liposuction, recontouring the cheekbones, perhaps a rib extraction or two, all finished off with breast augmentation" (164). In a similar vein, Young (1990b) notes that, while it is important not to criticize women who elect to have cosmetic surgery, it is "questionable" whether their actions can be construed as a "choice," and, indeed, she can't help but suspect that much of the cosmetic surgery that women undergo must be "frivolous and unnecessary, like diamonds or furs" (202).

12. I would like to thank Laurie Shrage for bringing this image to my attention.

13. The meaning of Helena Bonham-Carter's character changes as well. In the film, she is cast as a human-sympathizing ape in a world where apes have the power, and humans, doomed to slave labor, are facing extinction. The film emphasizes the similarity between humans and apes, endowing apes with all the attributes, good and bad, normally reserved for humans. While Bonham-Carter is praised for how her human thoughts and emotions "show" through her makeup, she becomes "just an ape" when pictured with Jackson. If her image "racializes" him, his image "de-humanizes" her, returning her unambiguously to the animal world.

14. In this sense, the desire to become "ethnically invisible" resonates with the wish to become "normal," "just like everyone else," expressed by the women I interviewed in *Reshaping the Female Body* (1995).

6

"My Body Is My Art":
Cosmetic Surgery as Feminist Utopia?

In August 1995, the French performance artist Orlan was invited to give a lecture at a multimedia festival in Amsterdam.[1] Orlan has caused considerable furor in the international art world in recent years for her radical body art in which she has her face surgically refashioned before the camera. On this particular occasion, the artist read a statement about her art while images of one of her operations flashed on the screen behind her. The audience watched as the surgeon inserted needles into her face, sliced open her lips, and, most gruesomely of all, severed her ear from the rest of her face with his scalpel. While Orlan appeared to be unmoved by these images, the audience was clearly shocked. Agitated whispers could be heard, and several people left the room. Obviously irritated, Orlan interrupted her lecture and asked whether it was "absolutely necessary to talk about the pictures *now*" or whether she could proceed with her talk. Finally, one young woman stood up and exclaimed: "You act as though it were not you, up there on the screen."[2]

This may seem like a somewhat naive reaction. Good art is, after all, about shifting our perceptions and opening up new vistas. That this causes the audience some unease goes without saying. Moreover, the young woman's reaction is not directed at Orlan the artist who is explaining her art, but rather at Orlan the woman who has had painful surgery. Here is a woman whose face has been mutilated and yet discusses it intellectually and dispassionately. The audience is squirming, and Orlan is acting *as though* she were not directly involved.

Given my research on cosmetic surgery, I was obviously intrigued by Orlan and the reactions she evokes. While I was fascinated by her willingness to put her body under the knife, however, I did not immediately see similarities between her project and my own, which was to understand why "ordinary" women

have cosmetic surgery. On the contrary, I placed Orlan alongside other contemporary women artists who use their bodies to make radical statements
about a male-dominated social world: Cindy Sherman's inflatable porno dolls
with their gaping orifices, Bettina Rheim's naked women in their exaggerated
sexual posings, or Matuschka's self-portraits of her body after her breast has
been amputated. It came as a surprise, therefore, when my research was continually being linked to Orlan's project. Friends and colleagues sent me clip-
pings about Orlan. At lectures about my work, I was invariably asked what I
thought about Orlan. Journalists juxtaposed interviews with me and Orlan for
their radio programs or discussed us in the same breath in their newspaper
pieces. Our projects were cited as similar in their celebration of women's
agency and our insistence that cosmetic surgery was about more than beauty.[3]
We were both described as feminists who had gone against the feminist mainstream and dared to be politically incorrect. By exploring the empowering possibilities of cosmetic surgery, we were viewed as representatives of a more nuanced and—some would say—refreshing perspective on cosmetic surgery.

These reactions have increasingly led me to reconsider my initial belief
that Orlan's surgical experiments have nothing do with the experiences of
women who have cosmetic surgery. In particular, two questions have begun
to occupy my attention.

The first is to what extent Orlan's aims coincide with my own, that is, to
provide a feminist critique of the technologies and practices of the feminine
beauty system while taking women who have cosmetic surgery seriously.

The second is whether Orlan's project can provide insight into the motives
of the run-of-the-mill cosmetic surgery recipient.

In this chapter, I am going to begin with this second question. After looking at Orlan's performances as well as how she justifies them, I will consider
the possible similarities between her surgical experiences and the surgical experiences of the women I spoke with. I will then return to the first question
and consider the status of Orlan's art as feminist critique of cosmetic surgery—that is, as a utopian revisioning of a future where women reappropriate cosmetic surgery for their own ends. In conclusion, I argue that—when all
is said and done—surgical utopias may be better left to art than to feminist
critique.

ORLAN'S BODY ART

Orlan came of age in the sixties—the era of the student uprisings in Paris, the
"sexual revolution," and the emergence of populist street theater. As a visual
artist, she has always used her own body in unconventional ways to challenge

gender stereotypes, defy religion, and, more generally, to shock her audience (Lovelace 1995). For example, in the sixties, she displayed the sheets of her bridal trousseau stained with semen to document her various sexual encounters, thereby poking fun at the demands for virginity in marriageable females in France. In the seventies, she went to the Louvre with a small audience and pasted a small triangle of her own pubic hair to the voluptuously reclining nude depicted in the *Rape of Antiope*—a hairless body devoid of subjecthood, a mere object for consumption. In the eighties, Orlan shocked Parisian audiences by displaying her magnified genitals, held open by means of pincers, with the pubic hair painted yellow, blue, and red (the red was menstrual blood). A video camera was installed to record the faces of her viewers who were then given a text by Freud on castration anxiety.

Her present project in which she uses surgery as a performance is, by far, her most radical and outrageous. She devised a computer-synthesized ideal self-portrait based on features taken from women in famous art works: the forehead of da Vinci's *Mona Lisa*, the chin of Botticelli's *Venus*, the nose of the School of Fontainebleau's *Diana*, the eyes of Gérard's *Psyche*, and the mouth of Boucher's *Europa*. She did not choose her models for their beauty, but rather for the stories that are associated with them. Mona Lisa represents transsexuality, for beneath the woman is—as we now know—the hidden self-portrait of the artist Leonardo da Vinci; Diana is the aggressive adventuress; Europa gazes with anticipation at an uncertain future on another continent; Psyche incorporates love and spiritual hunger; and Venus represents fertility and creativity.

Orlan's "self-portraits" are not created at the easel, but on the operating table. The first took place on May 30, 1987—the artist's fortieth birthday—and eight more have taken place since then. Each operation is a "happening." The "operating theater" is decorated with colorful props and larger-than-life representations of the artist and her muses. Male striptease dancers perform to music. The surgeons and nurses wear costumes by top designers, and Orlan herself appears in net stockings and a party hat with one breast exposed. She kisses the surgeon ostentatiously on the mouth before lying down on the operating table. Each performance has a theme (like "Carnal Art," "This Is My Body," "This Is My Software," "I Have Given My Body to Art," "Identity Alterity"). Orlan reads philosophical, literary, or psychoanalytic texts while being operated on under local anesthesia. Her mood is playful, and she talks animatedly even while her face is being jabbed with needles or cut ("producing"—as she puts it—"the image of a cadaver under autopsy which just keeps speaking").[4]

All of the operations have been filmed. The seventh operation-performance in 1993 was transmitted live by satellite to galleries around the world (the theme was omnipresence) where specialists were able to watch the operation and ask questions that Orlan then answered "live" during the performance. In between operations, Orlan speaks about her work at conferences and festivals throughout the world where she also shows photographs and video clips of her operations. Under the motto "My body is my art," she has collected souvenirs from her operations and stored them in circular, plexiglass receptacles that are on display in her studio in Ivry, France. These "reliquaries" include pieces of her flesh preserved in liquid, sections of her scalp with hair still attached, fat cells that have been suctioned out of her face, or crumpled bits of surgical gauze drenched in her blood. She sells them for as much as 1,500 Euros, intending to continue until she has "no more flesh to sell."

Orlan's performances require a strong stomach, and her audiences have been known to walk out midway through the video. The confrontation of watching the artist direct the cutting up of her own body is just too much for many people to bear. Reactions range from irritation to—in Vienna—a viewer fainting.[5] While Orlan begins her performances by apologizing to her audiences for causing them pain, this is precisely her intention. As she puts it, art has to be transgressive, disruptive, and unpleasant in order to have a social function. ("Art is not for decorating apartments, for we already have plenty of that with aquariums, plants, carpets, curtains, furniture."[6]) Both artist and audience need to feel uncomfortable so that "we will be forced to ask questions."

For Orlan, the most important question concerns "the status of the body in our society and its future . . . in terms of the new technologies."[7] The body has traditionally been associated with the innate, the immutable, the God given, or the "fated-ness" of human life. Within modernist science, the body has been treated as the biological bedrock of theories on self and society—the "only constant in a rapidly changing world" (Frank 1990, 133). In recent years, this view has become increasingly untenable. The body—as well as our beliefs about it—is subject to enormous variation, both within and between cultures. Postmodern thinkers have rejected the notion of a biological body in favor of viewing bodies as social constructions. Orlan's project takes the postmodern deconstruction of the material body a step further. In her view, modern technologies have made any notion of a "natural" body obsolete. Test-tube babies, genetic manipulation, and cosmetic surgery enable us to intervene in nature and develop our capacities in accordance with our needs and desires. In the future, bodies will become increasingly insignificant—nothing more than a "costume," "a vehicle," something to be changed in our search "to become who we are."[8]

The body of which Orlan speaks is a female body. Whereas her earlier work explored gender stereotypes in historical representations of the female body, her present project examines the social pressures that are exercised upon women through their bodies, in particular, the cultural beauty norms. At first glance, this may seem contradictory, since the goal of her art is to achieve an "ideal" face. Although she draws upon mythical beauties for inspiration, she does not want to resemble them. Nor is she particularly concerned with being beautiful. Her operations have left her considerably less beautiful than she was before. For example, in Operation Seven she had silicone implants inserted in her temples (the forehead of Mona Lisa), giving her a slightly extraterrestrial appearance. For her next and last operation, she has planned "the biggest nose physically possible"—a nose that will begin midway up her forehead. Thus, while Orlan's face is an "ideal" one, it deviates radically from the masculinist ideal of feminine perfection. Her "ideal" is radically nonconformist. It does not make us aware of what we lack. When we look at Orlan, we are reminded that we can use our imagination to become the persons we want to be.

Orlan's project explores the problem of identity. Who she is, is in constant flux or, as she puts it, "by wanting to become another, I become myself." "I am a bulldozer: dominant and aggressive. . . . but if that becomes fixed it is a handicap. . . . I, therefore, renew myself by becoming timid and tender."[9] Her identity project is radical precisely because she is willing to alter her body surgically in order to experiment with different identities. What happens to the notion of "race," she wonders, if I shed my white skin for a black one?[10] Similarly, she rejects gender as a fixed category when she claims: "I am a woman to woman transsexual act." However, Orlan's surgical transformations—unlike a sex-change operation—are far from permanent. In this sense, Orlan's art can be viewed as a contribution to postmodern feminist theory on identity.[11] Her face resembles Haraway's (1991) cyborg—half human, half machine, which implodes the notion of the natural body. Her project represents the postmodern celebration of identity as fragmented, multiple, and—above all—fluctuating, and her performances resonate with the radical social constructionism of Butler (1990 and 1993) and her celebration of the transgressive potential of such performativity.

For Orlan, plastic surgery is a path toward self-determination—a way for women to regain control over their bodies. Plastic surgery is one of the primary arenas where "man's power can be most powerfully asserted on women's bodies," "where the dictates of the dominant ideology . . . becom[e] . . . more deeply embedded in female . . . flesh."[12] Instead of having her body rejuvenated or beautified, she turns the tables and uses surgery as a medium for a different project. For example, when Orlan's male plastic surgeons balked at having to make her too ugly ("they wanted to keep me cute"), she turned to a female feminist plastic surgeon who was prepared to carry out her wishes. The surgical performances themselves are set up to dispel the notion of a sick body, "just an inert piece of meat, lying on the table."[13] Orlan designs her body, orchestrates the operations, and makes the final decision about when to stop and when to go on. Through the surgery, she talks, gesticulates, and laughs. This is her party, and the only constraint is that she remain in charge. Thus, while bone breaking might be desirable (she originally wanted to have longer legs), it had to be rejected because it would have required full anesthesia and, therefore, would have defeated the whole purpose of the project. Orlan has to be the creator, not just the creation, the one who decides and not the passive object of another's decisions.

ART AND LIFE

I now want to return to the issue that I raised at the outset of this article: namely, the puzzling fact that my research is continually being associated with Orlan's art. As one journalist noted after reading my book: the only difference between Orlan and the majority of women who have cosmetic surgery is one of degree. Orlan is just an extreme example of what is basically the same phenomenon: women who have cosmetic surgery want to be "their own Pygmalions."[14]

At first glance, there are, indeed, similarities between Orlan's statements about her art and how the women I interviewed described their reasons for having cosmetic surgery. For example, both Orlan and these women insisted that they did not have cosmetic surgery to become more beautiful. They had cosmetic surgery because they did not feel "at home" in their bodies; their bodies did not "fit" their sense of who they were. Cosmetic surgery was an intervention in identity. It enabled them to reduce the distance between the internal and external so that others could see them as they saw themselves.[15] Another similarity is that both Orlan and the women I spoke with viewed themselves as agents who, by remaking their bodies, remade their lives as well. They all rejected the notion that by having cosmetic surgery they had allowed themselves to be coerced, normalized, or ideologically manipulated. On the contrary, cosmetic surgery was a way for them to take control of circumstances over which they previously had no control. Like Orlan, these women even regarded their decision to have cosmetic surgery as an oppositional act: something they did for themselves, often at great risk and in the face of considerable resistance from others.

However, this is where the similarities end. Orlan's project is not about a real-life problem; it is about art. She does not use cosmetic surgery to alleviate suffering with her body, but rather to make a public and highly abstract statement about beauty, identity, and agency. Her body is little more than a "vehicle" for her art, and her personal feelings are entirely irrelevant. When asked about the pain she must be experiencing, she merely shrugs and says: "Art is a dirty job, but someone has to do it."[16] Orlan is a woman with a mission; she wants to shock, disrupt convention, and provoke people to discussing taboo issues. "Art can and must change the world, for that is its only justification."[17]

This is very different from the reasons the women I spoke with gave for having cosmetic surgery. Their project is a very private and personal one. They want to eliminate suffering that has gone beyond what they feel they should have to endure. They are anxious about the pain of surgery and worried about the outcome. They prefer secrecy to publicity and have no desire to confront others with their decisions. While their explanations touch on issues like beauty, identity, and agency (although not necessarily using those words), they are always linked to their experiences and their particular life histories. Their justification for having cosmetic surgery is necessity. It is the lesser of two evils, their only option under the circumstances. They do not care at all about changing the world; they simply want to change themselves.

Thus, cosmetic surgery as art and cosmetic surgery in life appear to be very different phenomena. I, therefore, might conclude that there is little resemblance between Orlan's surgical experiences and those of most women who have cosmetic surgery after all. Orlan's celebration of surgical technologies seems to have little in common with a project like my own, which aims to provide a feminist critique of cosmetic surgery. Consequently, comparisons between my research and Orlan's project can only be regarded as superficial or premature.

But perhaps this conclusion is overhasty. After all, it was never Orlan's intention to understand the surgical experiences of "ordinary" women. Nor is it her intention to provide a feminist polemic against the unimaginable lengths to which women will go to achieve an ideal of beauty as defined by men. Hers is not a sociological analysis that explicitly attacks the evils of cosmetic surgery and its pernicious effects on women (Lovelace 1995). Nevertheless, her project is an implicit critique of the dominant norms of beauty and the way cosmetic surgery is practiced today. It belongs to the tradition of feminist critique, which imaginatively explores the possibilities of modern technology for the empowerment of women. As such, Orlan's project might be viewed as an example of a feminist utopia.

COSMETIC SURGERY AS FEMINIST UTOPIA

Feminists have often envisioned a future where technology has been seized by women for their own ends. Take, for example, Shulamith Firestone's *The*

Dialectic of Sex (1970) in which she fantasizes a world in which reproductive technology frees women from the chores and constraints of biological motherhood. In a similar vein, the novelist Marge Piercy depicts a feminist utopia in *Woman on the Edge of Time* (1976) where genetic engineering has erased sexual and "racial" differences, thereby abolishing sexism and racism.[18]

More recently, the feminist philosopher Kathryn Morgan (1991) employs the notion of utopia to cosmetic surgery. She claims that refusal may not be the only feminist response to the troubling problem of women's determination to put themselves under the knife for the sake of beauty. There may, in fact, be a more radical way for feminists to tackle the "technological beauty imperative."

She puts forth what she calls "a utopian response to cosmetic surgery": that is, an imaginary model that represents a desirable ideal that because of its radicality is unlikely to occur on a wide scale (Morgan 1991, 47). Drawing upon feminist street theater on the one hand, and postmodern feminist theory, most notably Judith Butler's (1990) notion of gender as performance on the other, Morgan provides some imaginative, if somewhat ghoulish, examples of cosmetic surgery as feminist utopia.

For example, she envisions alternative "Miss" pageants in which the contestants compete for the title "Ms. Ugly." They bleach their hair white, apply wrinkle-*inducing* creams or have wrinkles *carved into* their faces, have their breasts pulled *down*, and *darken* their skin (Morgan 1991, 46). Or, she imagines Beautiful Body Boutiques where "freeze-dried fat cells," "skin Velcro," and magnetically attachable breasts complete with nipple pumps, and do-it-yourself sewing kits with painkillers and needles are sold to interested consumers.

These "performances" can be characterized as a feminist critique of cosmetic surgery for several reasons.

First, they unmask both "beauty" and "ugliness" as cultural artifacts rather than natural properties of the female body. They valorize what is normally perceived as "ugly," thereby upsetting the cultural constraints upon women to comply with the norms of beauty. By actually undergoing mutations of the flesh, the entire notion of a natural body—that linchpin of gender ideology—is destabilized.

Second, these surgical performances constitute women as subjects who use their feminine body as a site for action and protest rather than as an object of discipline and normalization. These parodies mock or mimic what is ordinarily a source of shame, guilt, or alienation for women. Unlike the "typical" feminine disorders (anorexia, agoraphobia, or anorexia) that are forms of protest where women are victims, Morgan's actions require "*healthy*" women who already "have a feminist understanding of cosmetic surgery" (45).

Third, by providing a travesty of surgical technologies and procedures, these performances magnify the role that technology plays in constructing femininity through women's bodies. At the same time, they usurp men's control over these technologies and undermine the power dynamic that makes women dependent on male expertise (Morgan 1991, 47). Performances show how technology might be reappropriated for feminist ends.

Morgan acknowledges that her surgical utopias may make her readers a bit queasy or even cause offense. However, this is as it should be. It only shows that we are still in the thrall of the cultural dictates of beauty and cannot bear to imagine women's bodies as ugly. Anyone who feels that such visions go "too far" must remind herself that she has merely become anesthetized to the mutilations that are routinely performed on women by surgeons every day (Morgan 1991, 46–47). Where the "surgical fix" is concerned, "shock therapy" is the only solution.

DOES COSMETIC SURGERY
CALL FOR A UTOPIAN RESPONSE?

The attractions of a utopian approach to cosmetic surgery are considerable. It enables feminists to take a stand against the cultural constraints upon women to be beautiful and dramatically exposes the excesses of the technological fix. It destabilizes many of our preconceived notions about beauty, identity, and the female body, and it provides a glimpse of how women might engage with their bodies in empowering ways. However, most important of all—and I believe this is why such approaches appeal to the feminist imagination—it promises the best of both worlds: a chance to be critical of the victimization of women without having to be victims ourselves.

While I am entertained and intrigued by the visions but forth by Morgan and enacted by Orlan, I must admit that they also make me feel profoundly uneasy. This unease has everything to do with my own research on cosmetic surgery. On the basis of what women have told me, I would argue that a utopian response to cosmetic surgery does not just open up radical avenues for feminist critique; it also limits and may even prevent this same critique. It is my contention that there are, at least, four drawbacks.

First, a utopian response discounts the suffering that accompanies any cosmetic surgery operation. One of the most shocking aspects of Orlan's performances is that she undergoes surgery that is clearly painful and yet shrugs off the pain ("Of course, there are several injections and several grimaces . . . but I just take painkillers like everyone else."[19]), or explains that the audience feels more pain looking at the surgery than she does in undergoing it. ("Sorry to have to make you suffer, but know that I do not suffer, unlike you."[20]) This nonchalance is belied by the postoperative faces of the artist—proceeding from swollen and discolored to, several months later, pale and scarred. Whether a woman has her wrinkles smoothed out surgically or carved in has little effect on the pain she feels during the surgery. Such models, therefore, presuppose a nonsentient female body—a body that feels no pain.[21]

Second, a utopian response discounts the risks of cosmetic surgery. Technologies are presented as neutral instruments that can be deployed to feminist ends. Both Orlan and Morgan describe surgery as conceived, controlled, and orchestrated by the autonomous feminine subject. She has the reins in hand. However, even Orlan has had a "failed" operation: one of her silicone implants wandered and had to be reinserted—this time, not in front of the video camera. Such models overstate the possibilities of modern technology and diminish its limitations.

Third, a utopian response ignores women's suffering with their appearance. The visions presented by both Orlan and Morgan involve women who are clearly unaffected by the crippling constraints of femininity. They are not dissatisfied with their appearance as most women are, nor, indeed, do they seem to care what happens to their bodies at all. For women who have spent years hating their excess flesh or disciplining their bodies with drastic diets, killing fitness programs, or cosmetic surgery, the image of "injecting fat cells" or having the breasts "pulled down" is insulting. The choice of "darkened skin" for a feminist spectacle, which aims to valorize the "ugly," is unlikely to go down well with women of color. At best, such models negate the pain. At worst, they treat women who care about their appearance as the unenlightened prisoners of the beauty system who are more "culturally scripted" than their artistic sisters.

Fourth, a utopian response discounts the everyday acts of compliance and resistance, which are part of ordinary women's involvement in cosmetic surgery. The surgical experiments put forth by Orlan and Morgan have the pretension of being revolutionary. In engaging in acts that are extraordinary and shocking, they not only entertain and disturb, but also distance us from the more mundane forms of protest.[22] It is difficult to imagine that cosmetic surgery might entail *both* compliance *and* resistance. The act of having cosmetic surgery involves going along with the dictates of the beauty system but is also a refusal—refusal to suffer beyond a certain point. Utopian models privilege the flamboyant, public spectacle as feminist intervention and deprivilege the interventions, which are part of living in a gendered social order.

In conclusion, I would like to return to the young woman I mentioned at the beginning of this article. At first glance, her reaction might be attributed to her failure to appreciate the radicality of Orlan's project. She is apparently unable to go beyond her initial, "gut level" response of horror at the pictures and consider what Orlan's performances have to say in general about the status of the female body in a technological age. She is just not sophisticated enough to benefit from this particular form of feminist "shock therapy."

However, having explored the ins and outs of surgical utopias, I am not convinced that this is how we should interpret her reaction. Her refusal to take up Orlan's invitation may also be attributed to concern. She may feel concern for the pale woman before her whose face still bears the painful marks of her previous operations. Or she may be concerned that anyone can talk so abstractly and without emotion about something that is so visibly personal and painful. Or she may simply be concerned that in order to appreciate art, she is being required to dismiss her own feelings.

Her concern reminds us of what Orlan and, indeed, any utopian approach to cosmetic surgery leaves out: the sentient and embodied female subject, the one who feels concern about herself and about others. As feminists in search of a radical response to women's involvement in cosmetic surgery, we would do well to be concerned about this omission as well.

NOTES

I would like to thank Peter van der Hoop for supplying me with information about Orlan. I am indebted to Willem de Haan, Suzanne Phibbs, and the participants of the postgraduate seminar "Gender, Body, Love," held at the Center for Women's Research in Oslo, Norway, in May 1996, for their constructive and helpful insights.

1. This festival was organized by Triple X, which puts on an annual exhibition, including theater, performance, music, dance, and visual art.

2. *De Groene Amsterdammer*, August 23, 1995.

3. See, for example, a recent article by Xandra Schutte in *De Groene Amsterdammer*, December 13, 1995, or "Passages and Passanten," VPRO Radio 5, November 17, 1995.

4. Quoted in Reitmaier (1995, 8).

5. *Falter* 49 (1995): 28.

6. Quoted in Reitmaier (1995, 7).

7. See Reitmaier (1995, 8).

8. Quoted in Tilroe (1996, 17).

9. *Actuel* (January 1991): 78.

10. Obviously, Orlan has not read John Howard Griffin's (1961) *Black Like Me* in which a white man chronicles his experiences of darkening his skin in order to gain access to African American life in the mid-1950s. For him, becoming the racial Other was a way to understand the material and bodily effects of racism—an experiment that was anything but playful and that ultimately resulted in the author's untimely

death from skin cancer. See Awkward (1995) for an excellent discussion of such experiments from a postmodern ethnographic perspective.

11. While Orlan has been cited as a model for postmodern feminist critiques of identity, her project is, in some ways, antithetical to this critique. She celebrates a notion of the sovereign, autonomous subject in search of self, which is much more in line with Sartre's existentialism than post-structuralist theory à la Butler. See, for example, the debate between Butler and others in Benhabib et al. (1995).

12. Quoted in Reitmaier (1995, 9).

13. *De Volkskrant*, June 5, 1993.

14. *De Groene Amsterdammer*, December 13, 1995, 29.

15. Quoted in Reitmaier (1995, 8).

16. Quoted in Reitmaier (1995, 10).

17. Quoted in Reitmaier (1995, 7).

18. See José van Dijck (1995) for an excellent analysis of feminist utopias (and dystopias) in debates on the new reproductive technologies.

19. Quoted in Reitmaier (1995, 10).

20. Statement given at performance in Amsterdam.

21. This harks back to the notion that women—particularly working-class women and women of color—do not experience pain to the same degree that affluent, white women and men do. This notion justified considerable surgical experimentation on women in the last century. See, for example, Dally (1991).

22. It could be argued that in the context of the art business, where success depends upon being extraordinary, Orlan is simply complying with convention. This would make her no more, but also no less, revolutionary than any other woman who embarks upon cosmetic surgery.

7

"A Dubious Equality": Men, Women, and Cosmetic Surgery

Reshaping the Female Body was about women's involvement in cosmetic surgery, based on women's reasons for having their appearances surgically altered. I linked women's specific experiences of embodiment to cultural notions of femininity and, more generally, provided a feminist analysis of the emergence of cosmetic surgery and its increasing popularity. My central argument was that cosmetic surgery cannot be understood as a matter of individual choice, nor is it an artifact of consumer culture that, in principle, affects us all. On the contrary, cosmetic surgery has to be situated in the context of how gender/power is exercised in late modern Western culture. Cosmetic surgery belongs to a broad regime of technologies, practices, and discourses that define the female body as deficient and in need of constant transformation.

Since the book was published, I have had the opportunity to talk to many different audiences—students, social scientists, philosophers, medical practitioners, consumer advocates, and feminist activists—and I invariably get the same response. They say: "What you have told us about women is very interesting. But what about men? Don't men worry about their appearance and want to look younger, thinner, and more attractive? Don't men have cosmetic surgery, too?"

My standard response and simultaneous defense of my "selective" approach to cosmetic surgery up until now has been to point out that, statistically, women are the primary targets of cosmetic surgery. Both numerically and ideologically, men as recipients of cosmetic surgery are the exception rather than the rule. They form such a small group that their importance for understanding the phenomenon of cosmetic surgery is negligible and, therefore, all but irrelevant.

However, in the past few years, it has not escaped my attention that there has been a small but steady increase in the number of men having cosmetic surgery. As of 1999, about 10 percent of the 2.8 million cosmetic surgery procedures in the United States were performed on men—that's 5 percent more than in 1992. Men had 83 percent of all hair transplants, 32 percent of all nose reshaping surgeries, 16 percent of all liposuctions, and 6 percent of all chemical peel procedures.[1] Although the percentage of men having cosmetic surgery still seems fairly small to me (with the exception of hair transplants), the media attention being paid to cosmetic surgery on men is anything but small.

The media in the United States and Europe abound with stories of how men, like women, suffer doubts about their appearance, agonize over their baldness, worry about their "beer bellies" and underdeveloped pecs, bemoan their sagging eyelids and worry lines, and dissolve into panic about the size of their penis (this is now called the "locker-room syndrome"). Reports indicate that men are currently spending billions of dollars on beauty products, gym memberships and exercise equipment, hair-color treatments and transplants, and, of course, cosmetic surgery. Once regarded as a practice reserved almost exclusively for women, cosmetic surgery has now become acceptable for men. According to a 1996 survey in the United Kingdom, 13 percent of British men admitted that they "expected to have aesthetic surgery at some point" (quoted in Gilman 1999, 343). Businessmen are increasingly having face-lifts in order to maintain their competitive edge, and middle-aged men look to cosmetic surgery as a way to match their aging bodies to youthful outlooks and lifestyles (Gullette 1994).

Commentators have suggested that it is just a matter of time before men have caught up with women as objects of the "surgical fix" (Gullette 1994; Haiken 1997; Gilman 1999). While the media applaud this development as a sign that men are (finally) casting off the yoke of ugliness and seizing their "right" to self-improvement, the critics are usually more skeptical. Mike Featherstone (1991), for example, views men's involvement in cosmetic surgery as part of the universal capitulation to the seductions of consumer capitalism. Margaret Gullette (1994) worries that men are falling into the same cultural traps that have been laid for women and that feminists need to form alliances with men. But whether men's involvement in cosmetic surgery is viewed as desirable or as cause for concern, the implication in *both* cases is that what we are seeing is a new trend. Gender differences in bodily experience, body practices, and cultural discourses on beauty and body alteration are converging in the direction of sexual equality. The gender gap is closing or, as Gullette (1994) puts it, "for good or ill . . . we're all together now in a new era of sex, age, and gender politics" (222).

I must admit that my feelings are mixed about this assumption of parity between the sexes in the realm of physical appearance. I find it difficult to see men as the new victims of the "beauty myth." I am doubtful that cosmetic surgeons—most of whom are men—will ever enthusiastically promote, let alone perform, surgery on members of their own sex. But, most importantly, I am uneasy about this discourse of equality. It seems to erase women's long and painful history of altering their bodies to conform with the cultural dictates of femininity, while, at the same time, it denies men's specific experiences with their bodies and the cultural meanings of masculinity in relation to cosmetic surgery.

Bordo (1993) has criticized the discourse of equality as part of a more general cultural tendency in Western consumer society to erase differences based on gender/class/ethnicity/sexuality or nationality. She argues that a homogenous or universal ideal is promoted in any discourse of equality, whereby individuals are presented as having the same desires, needs, and opportunities for giving shape to their lives. Contradictory or unsettling images of systemic oppression, inferiorization, exclusion, or racism are denied or kept within the safe boundaries of exoticism. As examples, she discusses the proliferation of ultrafeminine models in men's business suits, which are standard fare in advertisements today. Such images erroneously imply that women simply need to dress for power in order to get ahead, thereby ignoring real obstacles facing women in the overwhelmingly masculine world of big business. Similarly, representations of white women with their hair in cornrows or dreadlocks suggest playful experiments with ethnicity and "race," while doing nothing to transform the dominant white, Western ideal of feminine beauty. Indeed, such images help to sustain these ideals by implying that every woman is equally free to create her body, her self, and the life she desires, thereby effacing the inequalities in social position and historical circumstances that make hair dressing practices anything but commensurate (Bordo 1993, 254).

In my view, the new equality discourse on cosmetic surgery resonates with the process of homogenization and the neutralization of differences based on structured forms of inequality, which Bordo describes as integral to late modern Western culture. When men and women are treated as generic individuals with the same desire for physical attractiveness, it is assumed that they are both equally subject to the pressures of cultural ideals of beauty. And, consequently, cosmetic surgery can be presented as a *similarly* desirable (or undesirable) and socially acceptable (or unacceptable) way for both sexes to change their bodies, their identities, and their lives.

In this chapter, I take issue with the notion of sexual equality in women's and men's involvement in the practices and discourses of cosmetic surgery. To this end, I explore representations of the male cosmetic surgery patient in the media and in medical texts. Drawing upon contemporary theory on masculinity, I show why, contrary to popular belief, we have every reason to expect that cosmetic surgery is, and will remain, a predominately feminine practice.

MEDIA REPRESENTATIONS

In the early nineties, a British program called *Plastic Fantastic* was aired during prime time and adapted for viewers in most European countries. The program was immensely popular.[2] It consisted of thirteen weekly install- ments that covered the most common cosmetic surgery procedures (face- lifts, liposuctions, breast augmentations, and "nose jobs," as well as the more recent cosmetic technologies like laser surgery and chemical implants). The format was standard for the "infotainment" genre. There were shots of the operation itself interspersed with the surgeon explaining the merits and oc- casional side effects of the procedure. Patients were filmed talking about their motives for having surgery, waiting in anticipation of their operations, or explaining afterward how delighted they were with the results. Various "experts" (psychologists, beauty specialists, art historians, and journalists) gave their considered opinions about the psychological and cultural signifi- cance of cosmetic surgery.

The makers of *Plastic Fantastic* emphasized at the outset of the program that cosmetic surgery was of interest to both sexes. To illustrate this claim, they devoted three of the programs to men and cosmetic surgery: "The Very Best for the Man" (eyelid surgery and laser resurfacing for businessmen), "Flex Those Muscles" (pectoral implants), and "The Rocket in Your Pocket" (on penile augmentation surgery). In the first, the focus is on a baby-boomer generation of men in search of perennial youth and anxious to maintain its position in the work world. Businessmen are shown, earnestly assuring the audience that they want to keep "sharp" and "maximize their potential." Sur- geons warn, however, that surgical procedures often have a long recovery time, and there are frequently unpleasant side effects (like scars behind the earlobes following a face-lift, or eyes that tear up after eyelid surgery). In the program on pectoral implants ("Flex Those Muscles"), the recipients are male go-go dancers, bartenders, and fitness fanatics who want to take the "easy way." Experts remark that implants are a sign of "gym culture with a vengeance," and that men are frequently more "vain" than women. Many protest that they couldn't imagine having implants themselves, and they are scarcely able to disguise their disapproval at such "frivolous" interventions. The surgeons aren't enthusiastic, either, but, as they put it, "If we don't do them, someone else will."

In the third episode, on penile implants, the patients are not shown full face. Instead we only see their eyes, darting furtively around the room as each po- tential patient relates his suffering with his small penis. One of the two patients interviewed is of Asian descent, markedly "Other" in the context of the white British surgeons and patients presented in the other installments of *Plastic*

Fantastic.[3] The camera shoots his hands, wringing nervously in his lap, as he confides his traumatic locker-room experiences where he does not, literally, "measure up" to other men. While their reasons for wanting the surgery resonate with the reasons women give for wanting cosmetic surgery—feeling different, lacking self-confidence, being teased about their appearance—these men's presentation is so full of hesitation and shame that the viewer feels more pity than understanding. While the male "experts" describe the operation as "appalling," the female "experts" can't contain their laughter. They make jokes about "shrunken willies" and remark mischievously that "it's not the lead in your pencil which counts but how you write with it." As one woman put it, "You just can't take it seriously." The surgeons are almost unanimously negative about the surgery, exclaiming that it's "nonsense," "peacockery," or "positively a nightmare."[4] The emphasis is on side effects, risks, and lack of adequate knowledge. They are much more negative about penis augmentations than they were about breast augmentations.

While these reactions are—perhaps predictably—the most extreme with penile augmentation surgery, they suggest that cosmetic surgery, contrary to the current emphasis on sexual equality in the realm of body alteration, may not be quite the same kind of undertaking for men that it is for women. Take, for example, the episode in *Plastic Fantastic* on breast augmentation surgery (called " Fairy Tales of the Breast"). While the surgery is *technically* similar to the penile augmentation in terms of procedure, severity of side effects, and risks involved, it is represented in a very *different* way.[5]

The augmentation candidates are white women of different age groups and social backgrounds. They are introduced by name, and they are shown full face, explaining why they want the operation. Their reasons seem plausible, and their enthusiasm for the operation is so convincing that it is hard for the viewer not to take their point of view. Although some of the "experts" are a bit ambivalent ("I can't see myself doing it"), they remain basically nonjudgmental ("If that's what she wants, it's okay by me"). A male classical scholar—presented as a beauty expert—provides the clincher—that beauty has always been a concern for women; it is, therefore, only "natural" that women would want to have cosmetic surgery. The surgeons also seem to have no trouble with breast augmentations. They provide straightforward information about the procedure and emphasize its safety. Although the problems with silicone are still fresh in their memories, they downplay these dangers by noting new developments in implant technology (the use of soybean oil in implants rather than silicone).

Having watched and analyzed many similar television programs about cosmetic surgery, I believe that *Plastic Fantastic* is a typical example of the way in which the media portray the new trend of cosmetic surgery for men. On the one hand, cosmetic surgery is presented as just as relevant for men as it is for women. The viewer is warned not to believe that only women care about their appearance and try to do something about it. However, scratch the surface of this rhetoric of sexual equality, and one immediately finds an unmistakable ambivalence about men and cosmetic surgery. In their ambiguity, the reactions of the patients, experts, and surgeons on *Plastic Fantastic* suggest that cosmetic surgery is not quite the same kind of undertaking for men and women, after all. While the patients and experts seem to find it understandable and even "natural" for women to have their bodies altered surgically, a man who has cosmetic surgery seems uncomfortable or—in the case of penile surgery—deeply ashamed. Experts clearly regard him as, at best, ridiculous and, at worst, an aberration, someone who is different, deviant, or even pathological. The surgeons appear to embrace cosmetic surgery for women with enthusiasm—as essentially beneficial and unproblematic. Cosmetic surgery for men, however, is treated as a potentially dangerous and risky endeavor. For the surgeons on *Plastic Fantastic,* caution is clearly in order when operating on male patients.

These surgeons' reluctance may, of course, simply be an artifact of the media, reflecting a more general cultural unease about men having cosmetic surgery. Perhaps surgeons in real-life professional circumstances are more "enlightened" about performing their services on this new group of patients. My own experiences in talking to cosmetic surgeons would suggest that this is not the case, however. In personal conversations, surgeons have often expressed doubts about any man who would want to put himself under the knife for the sake of appearance. "I have trouble understanding these guys" or "They must have other problems, too" were frequently heard remarks. Surgeons also seemed more reticent than enthusiastic about trying out new technologies on men, expressing concern about the side effects and suggesting that "a lot more testing needs to be done" before "some of these operations" should be performed on men.

A case in point is the response of the medical profession in the Netherlands to penile augmentation surgery. It was heralded in the early nineties as a revolutionary solution to the problem of "locker-room anxiety." However, just two years later, it was discontinued. The reason given was that men were complaining so much about the results and side effects that the surgeons were worried about being able to give them the "proper post-operative care"! In the United States, penile surgery has also become controversial as practitioners increasingly face criticisms from their colleagues and costly malpractice suits from disappointed patients.[6]

In order to understand a surgeon's reluctance about operating on male patients, I shall now take a look at medical representations of the male cosmetic surgery patient. How do medical texts written by surgeons themselves portray the men who have cosmetic surgery? Are cosmetic operations treated similarly for both sexes, or do these texts display the same kind of ambivalence about men that permeates the media representations of cosmetic surgery for men?

MEDICAL TEXTS

In recent years, plastic surgery has begun to address the specific needs and problems of the male patient. For example, the well-known American medical journal *Clinics in Plastic Surgery* (Connell 1991) devoted an entire issue to male aesthetic[7] surgery based on a symposium on the same topic. Face-lifts, nose jobs, and liposuctions were presented as procedures that could be performed on both sexes. Cosmetic surgery specifically aimed at men's problems with their appearance (like hair restoration surgery, calf and buttock enhancement, or chin implants) was described as involving the same techniques and materials as cosmetic surgery for women. From a medical point of view, cosmetic surgery was depicted as the same for men and women. However, while the procedures and technologies were treated as similar, men and women as patients definitely were not.

Most surgical texts represent female patients as struggling with bodies that do not meet the cultural norms of feminine beauty. Surgeons believe that since women are taught to look good and disguise their real or imagined "defects," it can be taken for granted that a woman will want to look as pretty as she can (Dull and West 1991). Surgeons expect women to have "self esteem issues" when it comes to their appearance. Since medicine has historically defined the female body as deficient and in need of repair, cosmetic surgery is easily legitimated as a "natural" and, therefore, acceptable therapy for women's problems with their appearance.

In contrast, surgeons describe men as having cosmetic surgery for different reasons than women do. Men seek out surgery for "functional reasons" or "clear-cut physical complaints" rather than the "purely aesthetic reasons" put forth by women (Flowers 1991, 689). Or, they are concerned about minimizing serious "deformities," while women merely expect "a more attractive nose" (Daniel 1991, 752). Moreover, men do not like "sitting around in waiting rooms with women" and are much more reticent than women to discuss their problems publicly—that is, with a surgeon (Terrino 1991, 732). While some surgeons pay lip service to reports in the lay press that substantial numbers of aging businessmen are seeking cosmetic surgery in order to improve their prospects of professional advancement, they believe that additional justification is needed for men to easily accept the "concept of surgery for aesthetic improvement alone" (Flowers 1991, 691).

Although the "cultural barriers" to men having cosmetic surgery have been "crumbling" since the 1960s, men who desire cosmetic surgery still tend to be regarded with some suspicion (Haiken 1997, 155–61). In the medical literature, they are referred to as "overly-narcissistic" and "effeminate." As one American surgeon put it, "Any man considering a face-lift is probably an aging actor, a homosexual, or both" (quoted in Haiken 1997, 156). References are frequently made to bodybuilders whose desire for procedures is "fuelled by the fitness craze" (Novak 1991, 829), and case studies typically include "male beach-wear models" and "male hair-dressers" (Daniel 1991, 753–57). The before-and-after photographs that accompany descriptions of procedures frequently portray male patients of Asian or African descent.[8]

Terms like "delusional psychotic," "grandiose ambitions," "latent schizophrenic, and "suicidal" abound in medical texts about the male cosmetic surgery patient. As late as 1967, it was asserted that male patients who had repeat surgery were "nearly all mentally disturbed" (Haiken 1997, 156), but the suspicion lingers on that the male patient is psychologically unstable. In 1991, one author noted that probably 15 percent of all men seeking rhinoplasties were the victims of "severe psychological obsession" and should be screened out immediately (Daniel 1991).

The assumption seems to be that "normal" men don't care about their appearance, and, if they do, there must be something wrong with them. Men who want cosmetic surgery are not only considered sexually or racially "deviant" or emotionally unstable persons to begin with, however. They also apparently make difficult patients. They have less tolerance to pain, require more medication than women do, and are likely to become restless when having to lie still for long periods (Flowers 1991, 698). Surgeons complain that men are much more squeamish than women ("queasy about being touched") and have a tendency to faint at the sight of a little blood. As one surgeon put it, male patients are typically "just totally edgy, jumpy sorts of people" (Dull and West 1991, 61).

Male patients also have more unrealistic ideas about what surgery can accomplish than women do (Mladick 1991, 797), and they are notoriously less satisfied with the results of the operations. In the well-known and widely cited textbook, *The Unfavorable Result in Plastic Surgery* (1984), women are described as generally willing to accept even the most negative outcome, while male patients tend to display "emotionally malignant reactions" to surgical failures. In the view of one contributor, men become easily "fixated on the damaged organ" and relentlessly pursue further operations (Gifford 1984, 32). Operating on male patients is a problematic endeavor as it activates "homosexual conflicts, unconscious castration wishes, and fears of emasculation," with the surgeon assuming the "role of the persecutor . . . the prototypical and primordial castrating father of the patient's childhood" (Gifford 1984, 41).

As if this weren't enough to make surgeons feel ambivalent about their male patients, they must also worry about the dissatisfied male patient's tendency toward paranoia and aggression against the surgeon in the form of litigation, threatening postcards, or midnight visits to the surgeon's home. Disgruntled male patients have been known to become violent with, in at least one case, fatal results.

This particular case has been written up in *Aesthetic Plastic Surgery* (Hinderer 1977) under the title "Dr. Vazquez Añon's Last Lesson." It is the dramatic story of an unhappy male rhinoplasty patient who stormed into the office of Dr. Vazquez ("one of the most outstanding plastic surgeons of Spain" [375]), killing him and his two nurses. The author of the article gives a detailed account of the patient's pathological personality, his dysfunctional family background, and the surgeon's misguided belief that the fact that the operation was medically successful was enough to protect him from his patient's anger. As the author puts it, the lesson came too late for the hapless Dr. Vazquez Añon, but let it be a "warning" to the rest of us" (Hinderer 1977, 381).

To my surprise, I discovered references to "Dr. Vazquez Añon's Last Lesson" in numerous straightforward medical texts about cosmetic surgery. The case was cited as evidence—and, often it was the only evidence—for generalizing statements about "the propensity of male cosmetic surgery patients toward violence" (Alter 1995) to more oblique references to the "psychologically explosive situation" of the male rhinoplasty patient caught in a "total" and "terrifying" transference based on the "nose-penis relationship" (Daniel 1991, 751).[9] The message to surgeons who would operate on men is clear: do so at your own risk.

In conclusion, the medical discourse has historically displayed, and continues to display, ambivalence about men having cosmetic surgery. From a medical point of view, cosmetic procedures for men may be currently greeted with the enthusiasm warranted by any new advance in medical technology. But while surgeons echo the general cultural sentiment that men are just as entitled as women to make use of techniques and procedures for beautifying the body, they seem less enthusiastic about actually operating on men. Their reluctance is not only expressed in personal conversations; it permeates medical texts about cosmetic surgery. Surgeons distance themselves from men who have cosmetic surgery by presenting them as "deviant" (homosexual or ethnically "other"), obsessive about their appearance, psychologically disturbed, or even violent. It is, therefore, unsurprising that, while they may continue to operate on men, they do so with some misgivings. In order to explain the unease among surgeons about performing cosmetic surgery on men, we need to look at some of the cultural meanings associated with masculinity.

MASCULINITY

Contemporary theorists of masculinity like Bordo (1994 and 1999), Connell (1995), Dutton (1995), and Kimmel (1996) have chronicled the new trend toward viewing the male body as an object to be improved, altered, and beautified. Formerly hidden from sight, men's bodies are currently on display in magazines, television, and films. Mike Tyson, Sylvester Stallone (as Rambo), and the Marlboro Man provide powerful models for how the male body should look: bulging biceps, well-defined pecs, washboard stomachs, piercing eyes, and jutting chins.

While such representations of muscle-bound masculinity do seem to provide the impetus for many of the newer cosmetic technologies for men (like pectoral implants and body contouring) and may, indeed, shape some men's desire for cosmetic surgery, it seems to me that this is only part of the story. Masculinity takes many forms, and certain forms are more dominant or, as Connell (1995) would say, "hegemonic" than others.[10] In Western culture, it is not the muscular bodybuilder or the provocative male centerfold who is "hegemonic" and at the top of the hierarchy; it is Rational Man who embodies real power (Morgan 1993; Seidler 1994).[11] High-level executives in the corporate world, financiers, Pentagon military strategists, professors at Ivy League universities, or professional men in the upper echelons of medicine and law all inhabit positions of wealth and power that enable them to legitimate and reproduce the social relationships that, in turn, generate their dominance. The dominance of these men rests on the repudiation of all telltale signs of femininity and gayness in themselves and the capacity to represent themselves as a universal norm—the unquestioned and unquestionable standard against which all others are measured and fail to measure up. It is the fiction of a unified masculinity that generates a deep-seated fear of the inferior "Other" (i.e., women, but also men who are less deserving due to their class, sexual preference, ethnicity, "race," or nationality) (Connell 1995; Frosh 1994; Segal 1990; Young 1990a). Indeed, controlling other men may be at least as, if not more, important than controlling women. Homophobia and a keen sense of "competitiveness," combined with a "combination of the calculative and the combative" interaction with other men, seem to be the central features of masculine power of the "Rational Man" variety (Donaldson 1993, 654–55).

The male body sits on uneasy footing with the discourses and practices of this particular brand of "hegemonic masculinity." For masculinity, which is guided by the dictates of rationality ("mind over matter"), the body is, at best, irrelevant and, at worst, an intrusive obstacle to the more important activities of the mind. The body is something to be ignored, denied, or, at least, kept firmly out of sight. If the male body comes into play at all, it is as the performing body: the body that has everything under control, the body that "does" but is never, never "done to" (Bordo 1994, 288).

This raises the question of whether cosmetic surgery can be a way for men to meet the cultural requirements of masculinity. Is it possible for men to achieve a more "manly" appearance by having their bodies reshaped, just as women can become more "feminine" through cosmetic surgery? Given the meanings associated with hegemonic masculinity in Western culture, I would argue cosmetic surgery cannot "enhance" masculinity for men in the same way it "enhances" femininity for women for the simple reason that the very act of having surgery signifies a symbolic transgression of the dominant norms of masculinity.

First, men who desire cosmetic surgery distance themselves from the norm of rational masculinity as disembodied. By treating the body as irrelevant to the intentions and activities of the mind, this norm implicitly requires that the body and all its material or emotional vulnerabilities be denied, hidden, or transcended. The male cosmetic surgery patient is preoccupied with his body, however. His body—its appearance and the suffering it entails—is central rather than a peripheral concern. The act of having cosmetic surgery situates a man squarely in his body—a body that is no longer mastered by a detached and rational mind.

Second, men who admit suffering because of how they look display behavior that, in our culture, is coded as feminine. Women are expected to be dissatisfied with their bodies and prepared to go to great lengths "for the sake of beauty." Men, however, are not supposed to care about something as trivial as appearance, let alone show these feelings in public. The female body has historically been regarded as an object of desire, subjected to the admiring or critical male gaze. (Rational) men are the ones who look, the "desiring sexual subject rather than the "receiver" of the desire of another" (Bordo 1994, 288).[12] By expressing his unhappiness with his appearance and, thereby, allowing others to critically view his body as an aesthetic object, the male cosmetic surgery recipient crosses the border of what is considered acceptable masculine demeanor. He acts like a woman.

Third, men who place their bodies under the surgeon's knife lose control— at least temporarily—of their bodies. Patients are, by definition, passive objects of the interventions of the surgeon. Patienthood invariably requires a submission to the physician's authority and a resignation of will, both of which are at odds to dominant cultural norms of masculinity. In a culture where agency, power, and control are linked to masculinity, by becoming a patient, a man takes on attributes that are at odds with hegemonic notions of masculine power.

These transgressions are exacerbated by the fact that most plastic surgeons are themselves men. The profession of surgery is traditionally one of the most male-dominated branches of medicine. Not only are most cosmetic surgeons men, but the professional ethos of surgery resonates with many of the ideals of hegemonic masculinity in Western culture (see chapters 1 and 2). Surgeons are rational men of science who view the patient as a body, as an object for their interventions. The act of surgery requires the ability to act aggressively and without trepidation ("cut first, think later"). As Cassell (1998) convincingly demonstrated, surgery is a quintessentially masculine profession— a profession that is not for "wimps," but for "real men," for men with the "right stuff" (17).

The male cosmetic surgery patient with his admission of bodily inadequacy, his display of "feminine" behavior, and his voluntary waiver of control over his body is likely to evoke discomfort in the male surgeon, while similar behavior on the part of a female patient would seem normal, natural, or just part of "the surgical experience." By willingly adopting a position of powerlessness vis-à-vis another man, the male patient disrupts the myth of a unified (rational) masculinity. The male surgeon will not only have to perform an operation that—symbolically—diminishes his patient's masculinity; by operating on a male patient, he will inevitably be confronted with the frailty of his own masculinity as well.

In this context, it is hardly surprising that many male surgeons are reluctant to perform operations on male patients or are inclined to find reasons why cosmetic surgery is inappropriate for men in general. It also makes sense that surgeons attempt to alleviate their uneasiness by distancing themselves from their male patients and relegating them to the position of "Other"—that is, different, deviant, disturbed, and dangerous. In this way, the uncomfortable subject of the surgeon's masculinity and the (myth of) masculinity as disembodied norm is kept firmly out of sight and out of mind.

THE GENDEREDNESS OF COSMETIC SURGERY

The current media hype on men as the latest objects of the "surgical fix" is not simply a case of mistaken thinking. On the contrary, it follows from a discourse of equality that currently pervades late modern Western culture and, as such, has far-reaching and systematic ideological implications. Equality discourse neutralizes the salience of gender (and other categories of difference) for understanding how men and women experience their bodies as well as the specific cultural modes of embodiment that are available to them. Under the banner of the new sexual equality in the realm of beauty practices, it becomes impossible to grasp why cosmetic surgery seems like such a "natural" and unproblematic step for a woman to take, while it is a shameful and humiliating operation for a man, only to be undertaken at great cost to his sense of self and how others perceive him. And, last but not least, equality discourse erases the long-standing feminist critique of the gendered underpinnings of the contemporary cultural obsession with beauty. Cultural discourses and practices that render certain bodies "drab, ugly, loathsome, or fearful" (Young 1990b, 123) become obsolete and, therefore, irrelevant.

Even this brief look at how masculinity and femininity shape experiences of embodiment indicates that cosmetic surgery has very different meanings for men and for women. Surgical techniques and procedures for beautifying the body may seem to be gender neutral, but individuals' experiences of embodiment as well as their involvement with cosmetic surgery are deeply gendered. The considerable statistical discrepancies between men and women as cosmetic surgery recipients are merely a reflection of these gender differences. Although taboos against men being concerned with their appearance may be weakening, the day that men catch up to women in the realm of cosmetic surgery still seems far away. And, if forced to speculate, I would suggest that we may have more reason to believe that the present gender gap in cosmetic surgery will prevail rather than that it will disappear.

NOTES

The quotation, "A Dubious Equality," is taken from Mike Featherstone (1991, 179) and refers to the promotion of men alongside women as consumers in the marketplace. I would like to thank Anna Aalten and Willem de Haan for their constructive suggestions for earlier versions of this chapter. My thinking on men and cosmetic surgery was also greatly enriched by discussions with participants of the European Union project "Beauty and the Doctor. Moral Constraints on Changing Appearance," which was held in Taormina, Sicily, in September 1999.

1. Information from the American Society for Aesthetic Plastic Surgery.
2. In the Netherlands, for example, a help line was set up to field phone calls from interested viewers—of which there were nearly 200 hundred every week for the duration of the program. *Plastic Fantastic* has been aired on another network since the original showing.
3. The other patient is a white Anglo bodybuilder.

4. Interestingly, the exception is two Italian brothers who share a practice and conjure up images of the diabolical twin gynecologists played in a double role by Jeremy Irons in David Cronenberg's horror film *Dead Ringers*. This is the story of Irons's characters' obsession with a patient who has three cervixes (played by Genevieve Bujold). Their fascination with her anomaly ultimately leads to madness and murder. See Kapsalis (1997) for an analysis of the gendered underpinnings of this film.

5. Breast augmentations and penile augmentations involve relatively simple procedures. Breast implants are inserted through a small incision into the cavity behind the chest muscles. Penile augmentations entail severing a ligament at the base of the penis, shifting the root of the penis from the inside to the outside of the body, and re-suturing the ligament. While both procedures involve minor surgery, which can be done on an outpatient basis, they both have numerous side effects. Breast implant surgery can cause numbness, scarring, encapsulation of the implant, which is, at best, painful, and, at worse, can necessitate the removal of the implants. Silicone can "bleed" into the body, leading to even more serious problems like arthritis or immune disorders. While the problems associated with penile augmentation are less health threatening, they are, nevertheless, considerable and range from the nuisance of having to shave hair growing on the shaft of the penis to scarring to painful erections or the inability to have an erection at all. Based on the consideration of these two procedures, the conclusion could be drawn that, from a technical point of view, cosmetic surgery is gender neutral, involving similar procedures and equivalent side effects and risks.

6. The most highly publicized case was that of a Californian urologist, Melvin Rosenstein (known as "Dr. Dick"), who claimed that he performed 3,500 penile operations, accounting for 70 percent of all such surgeries worldwide (Taylor 1995). As Rosenstein became increasingly embroiled in lawsuits from patients who claimed that he had mangled or deformed their penises, the U.S. media had a field day. Rosenstein was finally forced by the Medical Board of California to stop advertising "risky surgeries," and in 1996, his medical license was suspended. See *Los Angeles Times*, February 17, 1996.

7. Originally, the distinction was made between "reconstructive" and "aesthetic" surgery. "Reconstructive" is generally used for surgery that restores function, while "aesthetic" refers to procedures that are regarded as medically unnecessary or "just for looks." While the distinction is blurry in practice, it has historically been the subject of ongoing strife within the profession concerning which kind of surgery was appropriately "medical" and which was the domain of charlatans or quacks. "Cosmetic surgery" is a more recent and probably the most popular designation for surgery intended to improve or preserve attractiveness (see Gilman 1999, 8–16).

8. This corresponds with my own experience watching plastic surgeons present slides of before-and-after surgical photographs. In one case, the surgeon announced at the outset of his talk that "men have cosmetic surgery, too" and then proceeded to show slides of women patients. There was only one exception—a man with dark skin and African features. See, also, Gilman (1991 and 1999) and Haiken (1997, chapter 5), who explore the connections between ethnicity and "race" in the development and deployment of plastic surgery techniques and procedures for aesthetic reasons.

9. There has been a long tradition within popular and medical thought of connecting the size of the nose to the length of the penis, beginning with Ovid's *"Noscitur et naso quanto sit habet viro"* through Nikolai Gogol's (1991) novella *The Nose*, whose protagonist Major Kovaljov wakes up one morning without a nose, symbolizing male castration anxieties and the general social dissolution of the Russian nation (Gilman 1995, 70–71).

10. Connell's notion of "hegemonic masculinity" is about dominant representations of masculinity—representations to which men aspire but rarely achieve. However, all men, even those who resist hegemonic masculinity (gay men, unemployed men, "caring fathers," male feminists), cannot avoid being oriented toward hegemonic masculinity. They must invariably negotiate their identities vis-à-vis dominant notions of masculinity.

11. Donaldson (1993) and Wetherell and Edley (1999) have explicitly criticized the association of hegemonic masculinity in Connell's work with the "hero"—the cowboy, the sports man, the action film hero. These "public figures" may be symbolically attractive (Donaldson) but do not represent what most people—men and women—admire in men (Wetherell and Edley). bell hooks (1992), while not referring specifically to "hegemonic masculinity," argues in a similar vein that the association of black men with sexual potency has served more as a foil for constructions of white supremacist masculinity than as an embodiment of masculine power.

12. Bordo (1994) gives a good example in her description of the locker room—the most masculine of all settings. Men open themselves up for extreme feelings of discomfort precisely because their bodies are on display, vulnerable to the sneaky peeks of other men. Men can easily imagine that they are being looked at in the demeaning way they themselves look at women. This is threatening because it places them in the position of passive object and opens up their bodies for critical scrutiny as not measuring up. When heterosexual men feel discomfort at being looked at, they are also exhibiting homophobia—a flight from attraction to and admiration of the male body (284).

Epilogue

In this book, I have explored cosmetic surgery as a cultural phenomenon of late modernity. From its onset as a medical specialty at the turn of the nineteenth century, cosmetic surgery has been intimately linked to discourses of gender. These discourses have shaped its technologies and techniques, its professional ideologies, and, last but not least, the objects of its interventions. After taking a look at some early manifestations of cosmetic surgery, I turned to more recent discussions about cosmetic surgery and the current beauty "craze." In particular, I discussed the difficulties facing practitioners and policy makers in justifying surgery "for looks" as well as how recipients defend their own decisions to have their appearances altered surgically. I also explored some of the ways cosmetic surgery has been taken up in popular culture as a seemingly neutral technology, enabling individuals to create the body of their dreams. Through the book, I took my own uneasiness with the erasure of embodied differences under the spurious banner of equality as an analytic resource in order to critically engage with cosmetic surgery and the contemporary cultures that have spawned it. And, I showed why arguments based on (masculinist) models of distributive justice, universal rights, and freedom of choice do not do justice to individuals' bodily experiences. Instead I have proposed an approach that takes embodied difference (collective and biographical), suffering, and individuals' agency in giving shape to their lives under less than perfect circumstances as starting points for thinking about the normative issues involved in cosmetic surgery. In this book, I have further developed my earlier position on cosmetic surgery (Davis 1995), arguing that as concerned critics we cannot afford the comfort of "correct line" thinking. There is no easy solution to the dilemmas evoked by the enormous expansion and popularity of cosmetic surgery and certainly no way to "just say no."

Having come to the end of my book, it is abundantly clear that the subject of cosmetic surgery is anything but closed. Cosmetic surgery has, if anything, become even more popular, and the need to find ways to deal with the moral complexity associated with cosmetic surgery has, if anything, become even more pressing. New interventions or new applications of old and familiar techniques will continue to be developed. As their promises become more sensational, they will undoubtedly attract the attention of the media, seducing more individuals to place their bodies under the surgeon's knife. One doesn't have to be a technophobe to worry about the consequences of this diffusion of innovation. In particular, the widespread use of cosmetic surgery to eliminate physical markers of difference will continue to attract more and more individuals, paradoxically exacerbating the injustices and inequalities that produced the desire for surgical alteration of appearance in the first place.

As a way of provisionally bringing to an end what appears to be an unending saga, let me take a look at one more application of cosmetic surgery: facial surgery to eliminate the physical signs associated with Down's syndrome, a chromosomal disorder involving intellectual disability. Individuals with Down's syndrome tend to have a distinctive appearance, which includes slanted eyes, a flattened bridge of a nose, underdeveloped ears, the protruding tongue, and a round, flat face.

Plastic surgery to alter the facial features common to Down's syndrome is relatively recent. The first operations were reported in the 1960s in the United States and have since spread to Western Europe (Italy, United Kingdom) and Israel (Edwards 1997). The sole purpose of the surgery is to eliminate the physical appearance associated with the syndrome (the "Down's look") and includes eliminating skin at the inner corners of the eyelids (epicanthal folds) to lessen the slanted appearance of the eyes, or building up the flattened bridge of the nose, correcting ears, inserting cheek implants, and suctioning out facial fat from the cheeks and under the chin to make the face look less flat and round. In some cases, the jaw is reconstructed and the tongue shortened and reduced in order to keep it from protruding, thereby causing drooling, breathing difficulties, and speech intelligibility.[1] The surgery has no effect on the symptoms of Down's—mental impairment or inappropriate behavior that may cause social stigmatization. It simply makes it less obvious that the person has the syndrome.

This relatively new form of cosmetic surgery raises many of the same issues that follow in the wake of any "new" surgical intervention, and it also highlights the controversial aspects of surgically eliminating signs of difference. While it resonates with many of the themes discussed in this book, it also evokes such discomfort that it compels me to take another look at the moral and political implications of new forms of cosmetic surgery.

FACIAL SURGERY FOR DOWN'S SYNDROME

On January 13, 2002, a British documentary film with the title *A Real Face* appeared on Dutch television.[2] It was about the use of cosmetic surgery to make the faces of individuals with Down's syndrome look more "normal." In true infotainment style, *A Real Face* depicts the surgical trajectory of several candidates for facial surgery—two preschool children, Georgia and Michael, and Peter, a forty-four-year-old man, all with Down's syndrome. The program follows the three recipients through the various stages of plastic surgery, provides detailed coverage of the operations, and ends several months after surgery when the results can be assessed. The parents are interviewed at length about why they want surgery for their children, about their hopes and about their fears. The children, oblivious to what is being decided, are shown playing with their siblings or other children, being examined by the surgeons, and, later, recovering from the operations. The parents are shown discussing possible side effects of the surgery with the surgeon, who does his best to reassure them. In contrast, Peter makes his own decision. He is shown going about his daily routines in his hometown. We see him having breakfast at the local café or singing Everly Brothers hits before an elderly audience in his community center and decorating his Christmas tree with his social worker. He is interviewed at length about his expectations and shown in consultation with a psychologist and a plastic surgeon prior to the operation. Members of the local community center and his social worker are asked to comment on his surgery, along with his surgeon, who all express their opinions (and objections) to his decision.

HOPES AND PROMISES

While the operations are technically the same, the normative issues surrounding operations for children and for adults with Down's syndrome are somewhat different.

Unlike other forms of cosmetic surgery, facial surgery for children with Down's syndrome is performed without the patient's consent. Georgia and Michael are too young to know what is happening; it is their parents who decide to have the operation. The parents are portrayed as concerned and loving parents. While they love their children and regard them as valued family members, they also want them to have a normal life. As Michael's father put it: "He shouldn't be deprived of the operation just because he's handicapped." These parents don't want their child to be treated differently, and they worry about how he will fare in school or in public places. By changing their child's appearance, he will be "less different," "more like a normal kid," "less likely to stand out in a crowd." While they acknowledge that the surgery is not going to change the syndrome itself ("they are always going to be slower than other children"), they still insist upon having it because they want to give their children "every opportunity to live a normal life." Although these parents seem highly critical of cultural prejudices against children who are "different," they see no other option than to take a pragmatic stance. After all, "it's harder to change society."

The surgeons underline how facial surgery will make the children look normal. As one surgeon put it, it will help us "look through the mark of deformity and see the *real* child within." Or, in a more God-like vein, "it's taking children out of darkness into lightness." The parents are shown sitting in front of a computer while their child's face is "transformed" into a "normal boy, just like his brothers." Considerable attention is paid to reassuring the parents that the surgery is safe and that the child won't suffer beyond what the surgeon calls "an amazingly low discomfort level."

This reassurance falls flat, however, in the face of the horrific postoperative images of the children. They are shown perched on hospital beds, confused and dazed. Their faces, swathed in bandages, are swollen, bruised, and bloody. The viewer can't help but feel sorry for them. The parents are clearly horrified by the state their child is in (Michael's mother scoops her child up and begins rocking him in her arms, crooning "Oh, my sweet, brave boy"). However, they put on a hopeful face, reassuring each other a bit too heartily that the operation has been a success and they can already see signs of the "new" face. Or, as Georgia's mother put it: "Sometimes you have to be cruel to be kind. I wouldn't want her to reproach me twenty years from now because I didn't have this surgery done."

Several months later, we see the children again, with faces transformed but—in one case—scarred and requiring further "corrective" surgery. One scene continues to haunt me. It is the image of the "new" Georgia, with clipped ears and reduced tongue ("no more drooling"), surrounded by her nursery school class. The implication is that the same children who made her life miserable with their bullying and teasing prior to her surgery are now presumably going to accept her into their midst. However, as viewer, I could not help but notice the little girl sitting directly behind Georgia who is gazing at her with such a nasty glint in her eye that I found myself wondering whether poor Georgia's problems had only just begun.

But if I was left feeling doubtful and uneasy about cosmetic surgery for children like Michael and Georgia, what about adults with Down's syndrome like Peter? Does surgery seem more promising and give rise to fewer moral qualms in his case?

At first glance, Peter seemed to me just like any candidate for cosmetic surgery who just wants to have a more "normal looking" face. "I'd like to get married, have kids, settle down, have my own home. That's it really." Although he dreams of looking like Don Everly, he admits, somewhat ruefully, that he'll never look like Mel Gibson or Roger Moore. "I know I won't look like that; I just want to look normal." While he also acknowledges that he'll be disappointed if his life doesn't change after the surgery, he is still determined to go through with it. "I want to," he says.

His reasons seemed no different than those I had heard in the course of doing my earlier research from countless women who wanted breast augmentations or face-lifts in order to look "ordinary," less "abnormal," "just like everyone else." Nevertheless, I discovered that it was considerably easier for me to take their desire for cosmetic surgery seriously than Peter's. The program, in fact, made it impossible to believe that cosmetic surgery could really help him have a more "normal" life. His acquaintances expressed nothing but disapproval about Peter's plans to have his face "fixed": "He still won't be normal, will he?" was a frequently heard comment. Peter's social worker, while clearly sympathetic to Peter's plight, was equally skeptical: "He believes he'll find a wife, but that's ridiculous, isn't it? That's not about how he looks; it's about his personality, what's inside, isn't it?" Peter is shown being interviewed by a psychologist who, through her cross-examination about his unrealistic expectations, tries to make it clear to him that little is to be gained by having surgery. Even his surgeon is ambivalent about doing the surgery and points out that "it's about society accepting people who are different, isn't it?" He admits that he doesn't really believe that the operation will have much effect on Peter's life and, I must admit, neither do I.

By the end of the program, Peter has had surgery on his nose and eyes. He's pleased with the result and confides that he's "more confident" now and that his mates have even invited him to the pub. However, the image we are left with is of Peter in his assisted-living flat, sitting at his kitchen table, still hopeful, but still very much alone. It is a disturbing reminder that no matter how much surgery he undergoes, he will never have a "normal" life.

The documentary is constructed in such a way that the parental hopes and medical promises of a normal life through cosmetic surgery for children like Georgia and Michael are shattered against the stark reality of Peter's life. A "normal" face will never allow individuals with Down's syndrome to "pass" as normal. For everyone who knows them—their families, their friends, their service providers—they will still be perceived as "abnormal," and no amount of cosmetic surgery will change that.

Like many BBC documentaries, *A Real Face* is laudable in its open-ended approach to the subject of cosmetic surgery for Down's syndrome. Rather than taking an ideological position, which either extols the virtues of such surgery or expresses moral outrage at its excesses, this film suffices with simply setting out the complexities of the problem. It compels the viewer to confront the limits of "normalcy," appreciate the hopes and expectations that cosmetic surgery awakens in parents and recipients, and then proceeds to dash them on the harsh realities of a world that has little tolerance for individual difference. It makes the viewer uneasy and ultimately leaves more questions than solutions. Our inability to see Peter as a knowledgeable and competent agent forces us to rethink the uneasiness that is sometimes masked in other forms of cosmetic surgery by the reassuring excuse of individual choice. The problem is relocated in us, the viewers. Our discomfort at the sight of differently embodied individuals and our desire for a speedy solution are exposed for what they are: *our* problem rather than the problem of the (abnormal) other.

It is, therefore, my contention that this documentary provides a glimpse of the moral and political complexities that accompany many of the newer surgical technologies. In the remainder of this epilogue, I will discuss these complexities and show how they make a critical response to cosmetic surgery in the future both more difficult and more essential.

MORAL DILEMMAS

Several years ago, the Hastings Center organized a meeting with bioethicists, social scientists, medical practitioners, and policy makers to discuss the ethic issues that may emerge through new "enhancement technologies."[3] In addition to some of the standard discussions about whether "enhancement" through medical means was justifiable at all, three kinds of issues arose—the problem of *unfairness* (how much suffering should an individual have to endure); the problem of *complicity* to norms, which are themselves "suspect"; and the problem of *inauthenticity* (or what kind of life is being enhanced?).[4] I will draw on these issues in order to make sense of the moral complexities as well as the discomfort that is generated by the cosmetic surgery for individuals with Down's syndrome.

The first issue concerns how much suffering a person should have to endure because of her appearance before she has the moral right to have the problem surgically fixed. Since individuals with Down's syndrome are already suffering from the disadvantages associated with mental impairment, is it fair that they should also have to suffer because they have the facial features associated with Down's syndrome? This argument is used by surgeons to justify the surgery and was echoed by Michael's father, who explains that it's not "fair to penalize his son just because he's handicapped." As he put it, the operation should be regarded as similar to "having braces put on."

As a viewer, I had no problem identifying with the parents' concern about their children's future. In Western culture, a high value is placed on intelligence and self-reliance, while cognitive disabilities are stigmatized. It was easy for me to imagine that parents might be worried about their children being bullied by other children or treated differently. And what parents don't just want a "normal life" for their child? In this sense, the parents' reasons for undertaking cosmetic surgery on their Down's syndrome children resonated with the reasons that are given by any cosmetic surgery recipient—the desire to be ordinary, "just like every one else." It might even be argued that they have a "moral duty" to provide surgery for their children.[5]

But the parents' desire to prevent their children from suffering is complicated by the image of Michael and Georgia, who do not seem to be the least bit perturbed by their facial features. In fact, they were portrayed as happy, sociable children who had no difficulties playing with their siblings or talking to the surgeon. If anyone was suffering, it seemed to be the parents. They were worried that their children would "stand out in a crowd" or that other people would "treat them differently." They seemed to be less motivated by their child's actual suffering than by their own embarrassment or discomfort at a mental impairment that was so visibly marked.[6] But if their reasons for having the surgery were somewhat unsettling, I became decidedly uneasy when these same carefree children were shown with battered faces after having surgery—surgery that they neither chose nor could understand. Despite the parents' protestations that this painful ordeal was in the child's best interests, it sometimes seemed to have been done more in the interests of relieving their own anxieties or feelings of failure. Thus, facial surgery on Down's syndrome children is complicated by the fact that the children may not even notice it, let alone suffer. It is the parents who either suffer or imagine how their children might suffer in the future.

The second issue concerns the *complicity* to a potentially harmful notion of normality. While most cosmetic surgery is aimed at "normalizing" appearance that is deemed abnormal in some sense (too fat, too wrinkled, too unfeminine, or too "ethnic"), making the features of Down's syndrome individuals look more "normal" seems more problematic. Why are the physical signs of mental impairment so disturbing that they need to be disguised? What makes mental impairment so socially unacceptable that parents might prefer to expose their children to the pain and discomfort of surgery rather than allow them to appear in public spaces? The parents and the surgeons all insist that society should be more accepting of Down's syndrome and that discriminatory stereotypes against the disabled need to be changed. However, they still insist on surgery as a pragmatic solution, thereby reproducing the same discriminatory social norms that they find problematic themselves.

What makes cultural notions of normality even more problematic in this case is the lack of agency on the part of the recipient.[7] While a woman who has a breast augmentation or a face-lift is also complying with cultural notions of normality—and some would argue that the pressures are so great that she hardly has a choice—we still can assume that she is a knowledgeable and competent actor. She will have some awareness of cultural pressures to meet a certain ideal body ("I know every woman wants to be beautiful, but . . ."). She will also probably make her decision by weighing the risks against the possible benefits of the surgery, reflect on her action, ultimately choosing between the lesser of two evils ("It may not be successful, but at least I will have tried."). While this doesn't make the cultural beauty norms any less disciplinary, it does make her decision to have cosmetic surgery a choice, albeit a choice made under circumstances that are not of her own making.

The problem with cosmetic surgery for individuals with Down's syndrome is that it is not possible to soften the problem of complicity to problematic norms with a reference to the recipient's agency. In the case of children, the parents decide for the child, and, as we have seen, it is not easy to regard their decision as strictly in the child's best interests. But even in the case of an adult with Down's syndrome, like Peter, it is difficult to see him as a knowledgeable and competent agent who is able to weigh the risks and benefits of the surgery and reflect on the repressive character of cultural notions of normality. One of the most difficult parts of the documentary for me was hearing how hopeful Peter was about the results of the surgery and then listening to the doubts expressed by his friends and by various professionals. Would Peter be able to assess the risks and benefits of the surgery, and would he be able to find ways to live with the disappointments of a less than successful surgical outcome? Would he understand that a new nose was no guarantee that he would find a wife, let alone be able to start a family? As well equipped as Peter had been to build a life of his own, I couldn't help but wonder how he would manage to sort through the false promises of the "surgical fix." Facial surgery on Down's syndrome individuals is clearly complicated by their lack of agency—a lack that makes the cultural constraints of normality seem more harmful because they are not the result of knowledgeable assessment or active engagement with the situation at hand.

The third issue concerns *inauthenticity* and what is being "enhanced" by cosmetic surgery. Debates about cosmetic surgery often center around the "natural body" and to what extent it should be altered through technological means. The fear that cosmetic surgery may be going "too far" goes hand in hand with the notion that appearance is a trivial concern in the broader scheme of things and that a life worth living is a life in which you accept the body that you have. Critics have, of course, responded that the "natural" body has always been a fiction and that cosmetic surgery is just part of a continuum of interventions that individuals routinely perform on their bodies in order to give shape to their identities and their life projects. In short, no big deal.

If all cosmetic surgery is directed at transforming the "natural body" and trying to "pass" as a younger, more voluptuous, or more svelte version of the original, then surgery on Down's syndrome adds a somewhat diabolical twist. What happens when the outer symptoms of Down's syndrome are removed while the "inside" remains the same? Does the creation of the illusion of normalcy help the individual to live a better life? And what is actually being "enhanced"? One of the most deeply disturbing aspects of this surgery is that it creates a gap between the "inside" and the "outside," producing the illusion of normality while leaving the mental "abnormality" intact, but invisible. In this case, a "normal" appearance will hardly allow the individual with Down's syndrome to "pass"—or, at least, not for very long. Even as I listened to the parents' hopes and dreams for their children, I was imagining Georgia or Michael at school and what would happen when their classmates discovered that they weren't so "normal," after all. I wondered whether their surgically reconstructed faces would make them more rather than less vulnerable to bullying or harassment. Social interaction requires ongoing identity assessment and display, with participants assessing one another and acting according to their expectations. Would Georgia's or Michael's peers be more or less tolerant of their slowness without the forewarning that facial features provide? I asked myself.[8] And what about Georgia and Michael? Facial surgery means that they, too, will have to live a lie, forced to measure up to their appearances (and invariably failing) or, what the Dutch call, "having to walk on tiptoe." What kind of life will that be?

As I watched the documentary, I couldn't help but wonder why we would want to live in a world where all signs of disability or vulnerability or bodily difference have been hidden. It seemed to fall into place with similar phenomena: the elderly being tucked away in homes, the handicapped in institutions, the poor in ghettoes. What are the lives of the "normal" like when they never, ever have to be confronted with persons who look and, indeed, are different? Is it possible to realize our humanity without ever encountering another person as Other?[9] Ultimately, the most disturbing aspect of cosmetic surgery for Down's syndrome was the confrontation it provided with myself and the culture of which I am a part. It showed me just how far Western culture is prepared to go to pretend that "we" are all the same, and it provided me with a chilling glimpse of how the world might look if all embodied differences were eradicated from public view. Encounters with difference provide an opportunity for reflection about ourselves and others, which is essential to our humanity. Without this, our lives may be less rather than more worth living.

EMBODIED DIFFERENCES

Cosmetic surgery has become a standard accoutrement of late modernity. As we enter a new millennium, new technologies (or new applications of old technologies) for reshaping and beautifying the body are developing in rapid succession, each one seemingly more effective than the last. Cosmetic surgery continues to be avidly promoted by the media as a desirable and trendy consumer product, which individuals increasingly perceive as a necessary requirement in order to live the "good life." As pressures to meet the cultural ideals mount, cosmetic surgery will continue to appeal to marginalized or culturally stigmatized groups as a potential avenue to assimilation, a kind of surgical "passing": the middle-aged can look young, unfeminine women can become voluptuous with breast implants, while feminine men can become masculine with penile implants, and the ethnically marked can look whiter and more Western. As a result, perfectly ordinary-looking individuals already perceive their bodies as so deficient and ugly that they feel that surgery is their only recourse for a normal life. The distinction between "normal" and "abnormal" appearance has already become fuzzy, as normal increasingly becomes conflated with the desire to embody an ideal (Hausman 1995, 56).

While these developments have already elicited considerable concern, criticisms have tended to focus on the risks and dangers of the procedures and the practice of cosmetic surgery itself, for example, whether patients have been able to make an informed decision, to what extent operations are really necessary or not, or whether they should be covered by medical insurance. Other critics—including myself—have tried to find ways to take individuals' suffering seriously, while, at the same time, resisting the cultural discourses of inferiorization that produce the suffering in the first place. While these criticisms have been important, the core question continues to be whether cosmetic surgery is morally or politically defensible at all or whether the only "politically correct" response to cosmetic surgery is condemnation.[10]

At the outset of this chapter, I introduced the example of facial surgery for Down's syndrome because it defies any knee-jerk response of the "just say no" variety. The moral complexity of this example makes, in fact, such closure an impossibility. One of the reasons I found the documentary *A Real*

Face compelling was that it made it so difficult for me, as viewer, to take up a definitive position "for" or "against" cosmetic surgery for Down's syndrome. There was no Archimedean vantage point for me to occupy from which I could dispassionately consider the phenomenon without bringing my own emotions, my experiences, my embodiment, into play. It left me rather with unanswered questions and more than a little discomfort. The usual legitimations concerning the elimination of suffering, choice, and a person's chances for a good life were unraveling before me, and in their place, I was being forced to think about my own response to embodied difference. This particular case made me stop thinking about the people who have cosmetic surgery or the practitioners who perform it or even the media that promote it and, instead, to start wondering why the world I live in prefers to disguise difference rather than to confront it in everyday life. It made me wonder what kind of world this is, what kind of person it makes me and those around me, and—finally—whether this is the kind of world I really want to live in. It seems to me that these kinds of questions and this kind of discomfort are what deserve our attention—as concerns that affect us all.

NOTES

1. There is some debate about whether tongue reduction is functional or cosmetic. While mouth breathing may be detrimental, the hope that the surgery will improve speech intelligibility has not proven well founded. Studies show that the operation improves the aesthetics of speech: that is, by preventing drooling, the child looks better when talking (see, for example, Leshin (2002) and Klaiman et al. (1988).

2. "*Dossier: Een echt gezicht—Plastische chirurgie voor mogooltjes*" (Dossier: A Real Face—Plastic Surgery for Mongoloids), RTL4, January 13, 2002.

3. This was part of a two-year project that was conducted at the Hastings Center, funded by the National Endowment of the Humanities, which explored the worries generated by new biotechnologies for the enhancement of human appearance and capacities. The discussion centered around cosmetic surgery, genetics, and psychopharmaceutical enhancement (Prozac, "smart drugs"). See Parens (1998b).

4. See the excellent introduction to the project by Erik Parens in which these issues are set out (1998a).

5. See Edwards (1997) for a rendition of this moral argument. It could be argued that it is the parents' duty to act on behalf of their children, particularly because these children are not—and probably never will be—competent to act on their own behalf.

6. See Olbrisch (1985) in which the author refers to the fact that children with Down's syndrome are frequently concealed from the public by their parents.

7. In a somewhat polemical, but nevertheless thought-provoking article, R. B. Jones (2000) compares facial surgery on Down's syndrome children to female circumcision—another form of surgery that is undertaken by parents who believe that

their child will be unable to function in her society without it. He advocates treating both practices as a form of child abuse.

8. A friend told me how glad she was her son looked like he had Down's syndrome. It's much harder on children who have the syndrome but look "normal." The bullying that they have to undergo is merciless and unending.

9. Levinas is one of several contemporary philosophers who has grounded his ethics in encounters with alterity. In his view, the only possibility for ethical activity occurs through the realization (and acceptance) of irrevocable difference. We need it to become truly human. See, Levinas (1979 and 1991). See, also, McKenny (1998).

10. For a good example of this kind of critical closure, see Morgan (1991).

References

Aalten, Anna. 1997. "Performing the Body, Creating Culture." In *Embodied Practices: Feminist Perspectives on the Body*, edited by Kathy Davis, 41–58. London: Sage.

Alter, Gary J. 1995. "Augmentation Phalloplasty." *Urologic Clinics of North America* 22, no. 4:887–902.

American Medical Association. 1996–1997. *Physician Characteristics and Distribution*, 1996–1997 edition. Chicago: American Medical Association.

Andrews, Edmund. 1861. "The Surgeon." *Chicago Medical Examiner* 2:587–98.

Anthias, Floya, and Nira Yuval-Davis. 1992. *Racialized Boundaries*. London: Routledge.

Appiah, Kwame Anthony. 1996. "Race, Culture, Identity: Misunderstood Connections." In *Color Conscious: The Political Morality of Race*, edited by Kwame Anthony Appiah and Amy Gutmann, 30–105. Princeton, N.J.: Princeton University Press.

Awkward, Michael. 1995. *Negotiating Difference: Race, Gender, and the Politics of Positionality*. Chicago: University of Chicago Press.

Bames, Otto H. 1927. "Truth and Fallacies of Face Peeling and Face Lifting." *Medical Journal and Record* 126:86–87.

Banet-Weiser, Sarah. 1999. *The Most Beautiful Girl in the World: Beauty Pageants and National Identity*. Berkeley: University of California Press.

Banks, Ingrid. 2000. *Hair Matters: Beauty, Power, and Black Women's Consciousness*. New York: New York University Press.

Banner, Lois W. 1983. *American Beauty*. Chicago: University of Chicago Press.

Bartky, Sandra. 1990. *Femininity and Domination: Studies in the Phenomenology of Oppression*. New York: Routledge.

Benhabib, Seyla. 1992. *Situating the Self: Gender, Community and Postmodernism in Contemporary Ethics*. New York: Routledge.

Benhabib, Seyla, Judith Butler, Drucilla Cornell, and Nancy Fraser. 1995. *Feminist Contentions: A Philosophical Exchange*. New York: Routledge.

Billig, Michael. 1987. *Arguing and Thinking: A Rhetorical Approach to Social Psychology*. Cambridge, U.K.: Cambridge University Press.

———. 1991. *Ideology and Opinions: Studies in Rhetorical Psychology*. London: Sage.

Billig, Michael, Susan Condor, Derek Edwards, Mike Gane, David Middleton, and Alan Radley. 1988. *Ideological Dilemmas: A Social Psychology of Everyday Thinking*. London: Sage.

Bordo, Susan. 1986. "The Cartesian Masculination of Thought." *Signs* 11:439–56.

———. 1987. *The Flight to Objectivity: Essays on Cartesianism and Culture*. Albany, N.Y.: SUNY Press.

———. 1993. *Unbearable Weight: Feminism, Western Culture, and the Body*. Berkeley: University of California Press.

———. 1994. "Reading the Male Body." In *The Male Body*, edited by Laurence Goldstein, 265–306. Ann Arbor: Michigan University Press.

———. 1997. *Twilight Zones: The Hidden Life of Cultural Images from Plato to O. J.* Berkeley: University of California Press.

———. 1999. *The Male Body*. New York: Farrar, Straus & Giroux.

Bouman, F. G. 1975. "De vorm een functie: 25 jaar plastische en reconstructieve chirurgie als specialism in Nederland." ("The Form as Function: 25 Years of Plastic and Reconstructive Surgery as Specialty in the Netherlands.") Inaugural address at the Faculty of Medicine, Free University, Amsterdam, Netherlands.

Bourguet, Julien. 1928. "Notre traitement chirurgical de 'poches' sous les yeux sans cicatrice." *Archives Franco-Belges de Chirurgie* 31:133–37.

Boxer, Marilyn J. 1982. "'First Wave' Feminism in Nineteenth-Century France: Class, Family and Religion." *Women's Studies International Forum* 5, no. 6:551–59.

Brah, Avtar. 1996. *Cartographies of Diaspora: Contesting Identities*. London: Routledge.

Brodzki, Bella, and Celeste Schenck, eds. 1988. *Life Lines: Theorizing Women's Autobiography*. Ithaca, N.Y.: Cornell University Press.

Butler, Judith. 1990. *Gender Trouble: Feminism and the Subversion of Identity*. New York: Routledge.

———. 1993. *Bodies That Matter: On the Discursive Limits of "Sex."* New York: Routledge.

Carroll, Noël. 2000. "Ethnicity, Race, and Monstrosity: The Rhetorics of Horror and Humor." In *Beauty Matters*, edited by Peg Zeglin Brand, 37–56. Bloomington: Indiana University Press.

Cassell, Joan. 1984. *Expected Miracles: Surgeons at Work*. Philadelphia: Temple University Press.

———. 1998. *The Woman in the Surgeon's Body*. Cambridge, Mass.: Harvard University Press.

Chancer, Lynn S. 1998. *Reconcilable Differences: Confronting Beauty, Pornography, and the Future of Feminism*. Berkeley: University of California Press.

Chodorow, Nancy. 1978. *The Reproduction of Mothering*. Berkeley: University of California Press.

——. 1989. *Feminism and Psychoanalytic Theory*. New Haven, Conn.: Yale University Press.

Code, Lorraine. 1991. *What Can She Know? Feminist Theory and the Construction of Knowledge*. Ithaca, N.Y.: Cornell University Press.

Connell, Bruce, ed. 1991. "Male Aesthetic Surgery." *Clinics in Plastic Surgery* 18, no. 4:653–890.

Connell, Robert W. 1995. *Masculinities*. Berkeley: University of California Press.

Dally, Ann. 1991. *Women under the Knife*. London: Hutchinson Radius.

Daniel, Rollin K. 1991. "Rhinoplasty and the Male Patient." *Clinics in Plastic Surgery* 18, no. 4:751–61.

Davis, Kathy. 1988. *Power Under the Microscope*. Dordrecht, Netherlands: Forum.

——. 1991. "Remaking the She-Devil: A Critical Look at Feminist Approaches to Beauty." *Hypatia* 6, no. 2:21–43.

——. 1995. *Reshaping the Female Body: The Dilemma of Cosmetic Surgery*. New York: Routledge.

——. 1997. "Embody-ing Theory: Beyond Modernist and Postmodernist Readings of the Body." In *Embodied Practices: Feminist Perspectives on the Body*, edited by Kathy Davis, 1–23. London: Sage.

——, ed. 1997. *Embodied Practices: Feminist Perspectives on the Body*. London: Sage.

Dellinger, Kirsten, and Christine L. Williams. 1997. "Makeup at Work: Negotiating Appearance Rules in the Workplace." *Gender & Society* 11, no. 2:151–77.

Denzin, Norman K. 1989. *Interpretive Biography*. Newbury Park, Calif.: Sage.

Donaldson, Mike. 1993. "What Is Hegemonic Masculinity?" *Theory and Society* 22:643–57.

Dull, Diana, and Candace West. 1991. "Accounting for Cosmetic Surgery: The Accomplishment of Gender." *Social Problems* 38, no. 1:54–70.

Dutton, Kenneth R. 1995. *The Perfectible Body*. New York: Continuum, 1995.

Edwards, Steven D. 1997. "Plastic Surgery and Individuals with Down's Syndrome." In *In the Eye of the Beholder: Ethics and Medical Change of Appearance*, edited by Inez de Beaufort, Medard Hilhorst, and Soren Holm, 26–33. Oslo: Scandinavian University Press.

Ehrenreich, Barbara, and Deirdre English. 1979. *For Her Own Good*. London: Pluto.

Featherstone, Mike. 1991. "The Body in Consumer Culture." In *The Body*, edited by Mike Featherstone, Mike Hepworth, and Bryan S. Turner, 170–96. London: Sage.

Firestone, Shulamith. 1970. *The Dialectic of Sex: The Case for Feminist Revolution*. New York: Bantam.

Flax, Jane. 1990. *Thinking Fragments: Psychoanalysis, Feminism, and Postmodernism in the Contemporary West*. Berkeley: University of California Press.

Flowers, Robert S. 1991. "Periorbital Aesthetic Surgery for Men." *Clinics in Plastic Surgery* 18, no. 4:689–729.

Foucault, Michel. 1973. *Madness and Civilization: A History of Insanity in the Age of Reason*. New York: Vintage.

———. 1975. *The Birth of the Clinic: An Archaeology of Medical Perception*. New York: Vintage.

———. 1979. *Discipline and Punish: The Birth of the Prison*. New York: Vintage.

———. 1980. *Power/Knowledge: Selected Interviews and Other Writings, 1972–1977*. New York: Pantheon.

Frank, Arthur. 1990. "Bringing Bodies Back In: A Decade Review." *Theory, Culture & Society* 7:131–62.

Frankford, David. 1998. "The Treatment/Enhancement Distinction as an Armament in the Policy Wars." In *Enhancing Human Traits: Ethical and Social Implications*, edited by Erik Parens, 70–94. Washington, D.C.: Georgetown University Press.

Fraser, Nancy. 1989. *Unruly Practices*. Cambridge, Mass.: Polity.

Freud, Sigmund. 1909. "Der Wahn und die Träume in W. Jensens 'Gradiva.'" *Gesammelte Werke* 7:31–125. London: Imago.

Frosh, Stephen. 1994. *Sexual Difference, Masculinity & Psychoanalysis*. New York: Routledge.

Garfinkel, Harold. 1967. *Studies in Ethnomethodology*. Englewood Cliffs, N.J.: Prentice-Hall.

Gergen, Kenneth J., and Mary M. Gergen. 1988. "Narrative and the Self as Relationship." Vol. 21 of *Advances in Experimental Social Psychology*, edited by L. Berkowitz, 17–56. New York: Academic.

Gergen, Mary M., and Kenneth J. Gergen. 1993. "Narratives of the Gendered Body in Popular Autobiography." In *The Narrative Study of Lives*, edited by Ruthellen Josselson and Amia Lieblich, 191–218. Newbury Park, Calif.: Sage.

Giddens, Anthony. 1976. *New Rules of Sociological Method*. London: Hutchinson.

———. 1984. *The Constitution of Society*. Cambridge, Mass.: Polity.

Gifford, Sanford. 1984. "Cosmetic Surgery and Personality Change: A Review and Some Clinical Observations." In *The Unfavorable Result in Plastic Surgery*, edited by Robert M. Goldwyn, 21–43. Boston: Little, Brown.

Gilligan, Carol. 1982. *In A Different Voice: Psychological Theory and Women's Development*. Cambridge, Mass.: Harvard University Press.

Gilman, Sander. 1991. *The Jew's Body*. New York: Routledge.

———. 1995. *Picturing Health and Illness*. Baltimore, Md.: Johns Hopkins University Press.

———. 1998. *Creating Beauty to Cure the Soul*. Durham, N.C.: Duke University Press.

———. 1999. *Making the Body Beautiful*. Princeton, N.J.: Princeton University Press.

Ginsberg, Elaine K. 1996. "Introduction: The Politics of Passing." In *Passing and the Fictions of Identity*, edited by Elaine K. Ginsberg, 1–18. Durham, N.C.: Duke University Press.

Gogol, Nikolai. 1991. *Diary of a Madman and Other Stories*. Translated by Ronald Wilks. London: Penguin.

Goldberg, David, ed. 1990. *Anatomy of Racism*. Minneapolis: University of Minnesota Press.

Goldwyn, Robert M., ed. 1984. *The Unfavorable Result in Plastic Surgery*. 2d ed. Boston: Little, Brown.

González-Ulloa, Mario. 1985. "The History of Rhytidectomy." In *The Creation of Aesthetic Plastic Surgery*, edited by Mario González-Ulloa, 41–86. New York: Springer-Verlag.

———, ed. 1985. *The Creation of Aesthetic Plastic Surgery*. New York: Springer-Verlag.

Gorney, Mark. 1998. "Patient Selection for Aesthetic Surgery in the Non-Caucasian: Practical Guidelines." In *Ethnic Considerations in Facial Aesthetic Surgery*, edited by W. E. Matory Jr., 3–9. Philadelphia: Lippincott-Raven.

Gould, Stephen J. 1981. *The Mismeasure of Man*. New York: Norton.

Griffin, John Howard. 1961. *Black Like Me*. New York: Signet.

Gubar, Susan. 1997. *Racechanges: White Skin, Black Face in American Culture*. New York: Oxford University Press.

Gullette, Margaret Morganroth. 1994. "All Together Now: The New Sexual Politics of Midlife Bodies." In *The Male Body*, edited by Lawrence Goldstein, 221–47. Ann Arbor: Michigan University Press.

Haiken, Elizabeth. 1997. *Venus Envy: A History of Cosmetic Surgery*. Baltimore, Md.: Johns Hopkins University Press.

Haraway, Donna J. 1991. *Simians, Cyborgs, and Women: The Reinvention of Nature*. London: Free Association Books.

———. 1997. *Modest Witness@Second_Millennium. FemaleMan_Meets_OncoMouse: Feminism and Technoscience*. New York: Routledge.

Harding, Sandra, ed. 1993. *The "Racial" Economy of Science: Toward a Democratic Future*. Bloomington: Indiana University Press.

Hausman, Bernice L. 1995. *Changing Sex: Transsexualism, Technology, and the Idea of Gender*. Durham, N.C.: Duke University Press.

Haywood, Janet. 1985. *The History of Soroptimist International*. Cambridge, U.K.: Soroptimist International.

Hearn, Jeff. 1987. *The Gender of Oppression: Men, Masculinity, and the Critique of Marxism*. Brighton, U.K.: Wheatsheaf Books.

Hinderer, Ulrich T. 1977. "Dr. Vazquez Añon's Last Lesson." *Aesthetic Plastic Surgery* 2:375–82.

Holländer, Eugen. 1932. "Plastische (kosmetische) Operation: Kritische Darstellung ihres gegenwärtigen Standes." In *Neue Deutsche Klinik*, edited by G. Klemperer and F. Klemperer, 1–17. Berlin: Urban and Schwarzenberg.

Hollway, Wendy. 1984. "Gender Difference and the Production of Subjectivity." In *Changing the Subject*, edited by Julian Henriques, Wendy Hollway, Cathy Urwin, Couze Venn, and Valerie Walkerdine, 227–63. London: Methuen.

hooks, bell. 1990. *Yearning: Race, Gender, and Cultural Politics*. Boston: South End Press.

———. 1992. *Black Looks*. Boston: South End Press.

———. 1994. *Outlaw Culture: Resisting Representations*. New York: Routledge.

Jacobson, Nora. 2000. *Cleavage: Technology, Controversy and the Ironies of the Man-made Breast*. New Brunswick, N.J.: Rutgers University Press.

Jacobus, Mary, Evelyn Fox Keller, and Sally Shuttleworth, eds. 1990. *Body/Politics: Women and the Discourses of Science*. New York: Routledge.

Jacquemin, Jeannine. 1988. *Suzanne Noël*. Paris: Soroptimist International.

Jones, R. B. 2000. "Parental Consent to Cosmetic Facial Surgery in Down's Syndrome." *Journal of Medical Ethics* 26:101–2.

Kapsalis, Terri. 1997. *Public Privates: Performing Gynecology from Both Ends of the Speculum.* Durham, N.C.: Duke University Press.

Kaw, Eugenia. 1993. "Medicalization of Racial Features: Asian American Women and Cosmetic Surgery." *Medical Anthropology Quarterly* 7, no. 1:74–89.

———. 1994. "'Opening' Faces: The Politics of Cosmetic Surgery and Asian American Women." In *Many Mirrors: Body Image and Social Relations*, edited by Nicole Sault, 241–65. New Brunswick, N.J.: Rutgers University Press.

Keller, Evelyn Fox. 1983. *A Feeling for the Organism: The Life and Work of Barbara McClintock.* New York: Freeman.

Kimmel, Michael. 1996. *Manhood in America: A Cultural History.* New York: Free Press.

Klaiman, P. et al. 1988. "Changes in Aesthetic Appearance and Intelligibility of Speech after Partial Glossectomy in Patients with Down Syndrome." *Plastic and Reconstructive Surgery* 82:403–8.

Klinge, Ineke. 1997. "Female Bodies and Brittle Bones: Medical Interventions in Osteoporosis." In *Embodied Practices: Feminist Perspectives on the Body*, edited by Kathy Davis, 59–72. London: Sage.

Lacqueur, Thomas. 1990. *Making Sex: Body and Gender from the Greeks to Freud.* Cambridge, Mass.: Harvard University Press.

Leshin, Len. 2002. "Plastic Surgery in Children with Down Syndrome." *Down Syndrome Health Issues*. http://www.ds-health.com/psurg.htm (last accessed April 5, 2002).

Levinas, Emmanuel. 1979. *Totality and Infinity: As Essay on Exteriority.* The Hague: M. Nijhoff.

———. 1991. *Otherwise than Being or Beyond Essence.* Dordrecht, Netherlands: Kluwer Academic Publishers.

Little, Margaret Olivia. 1998. "Cosmetic Surgery, Suspect Norms, and the Ethics of Complicity." In *Enhancing Human Traits: Ethical and Social Implications,* edited by Erik Parens, 162–176. Washington, D.C.: Georgetown University Press.

Lovelace, Cary. 1995. "Orlan: Offensive Acts." *Performing Arts Journal* 49:13–25.

Lury, Celia. 2000. "The United Colors of Diversity: Essential and Inessential Culture." In *Global Nature, Global Culture*, edited by Sarah Fanklin, Celia Lury, and Jackie Stacey, 146–87. London: Sage.

MacCannell, Dean, and Juliet Flower MacCannell. 1987. "The Beauty System." In *The Ideology of Conduct*, edited by Nancy Armstrong and Leonard Tennenhouse, 206–38. New York: Methuen.

McDowell, Frank. 1978. "Plastic Surgery in the Twentieth Century." *Annals of Plastic Surgery* 1:217–20.

———. 1985. "History of Rhinoplasty." In *The Creation of Aesthetic Plastic Surgery*, edited by Mario González-Ulloa, 87–114. New York: Springer-Verlag.

McKenny, Gerald P. 1998. "Enhancements and the Ethical Significance of Vulnerability." In *Enhancing Human Traits: Ethical and Social Implications*, edited by Erik Parens, 222–37. Washington, D.C.: Georgetown University Press.

McNay, Lois. 2000. *Gender and Agency: Reconfiguring the Subject in Feminist and Social Theory*. Cambridge, Mass.: Polity.

Maltz, Maxwell. 1954. *Doctor Pygmalion: The Autobiography of a Plastic Surgeon*. London: Museum Press.

Mama, Amina. 1995. *Beyond the Masks: Race, Gender and Subjectivity*. New York: Routledge.

Martin, Emily. 1987. *The Woman in the Body: A Cultural Analysis of Reproduction*. Boston: Beacon.

———, ed. 1998. *Ethnic Considerations in Facial Aesthetic Surgery*. Philadelphia: Lippincott-Raven.

Matory, W. Earle Jr. 1998. Preface to *Ethnic Considerations in Facial Aesthetic Surgery*, edited by W. Earle Matory Jr., xix–xx. Philadelphia: Lippincott-Raven.

Mercer, Kobena. 1994. *Welcome to the Jungle*. New York and London: Routledge.

———. 1997. "Black Hair/Style Politics." In *The Subcultures Reader*, edited by Ken Gelder and Sarah Thornton, 420–35. London: Routledge.

Miller, Charles Conrad. 1923. *Rubber and Gutta Percha Injections*. Chicago: Oak.

———. 1925. *Cosmetic Surgery: The Correction of Featural Imperfections*. Philadelphia: F. A. Davis.

Ministery of Health, Education, and Welfare. 1992. *Choices in Health Care*. Rijswijk, Netherlands: Ministery of Health, Education, and Welfare.

Mladick, Richard A. 1991. "Male Body Contouring." *Clinics in Plastic Surgery* 18, no. 4:797–822.

Morantz-Sanchez, Regina Markell. 1985. *Sympathy & Science: Women Physicians in American Medicine*. New York: Oxford University Press.

Morgan, David H. J. 1981. "Men, Masculinity and the Process of Sociological Enquiry." In *Doing Feminist Research*, edited by Helen Roberts, 83–113. London: Routledge & Kegan Paul.

———. 1992. *Discovering Men*. New York: Routledge.

———. 1993. "'You Too Can Have a Body Like Mine': Reflections on the Male Body and Masculinities." In *Body Matters*, edited by Sue Scott and David Morgan, 69–88. Washington, D.C.: Falmer Press.

Morgan, Kathryn Pauly. 1991. "Women and the Knife: Cosmetic Surgery and the Colonalization of Women's Bodies." *Hypatia* 6, no. 3:25–53.

Newton, Stella Mary. 1974. *Health, Art and Reason: Dress Reformers of the 19th Century*. London: John Murray.

Noël, Suzanne. 1932. *Die Aesthetische Chirurgie und ihre soziale Bedeutung*. Translated from the French by A. Hardt. Leipzig: Johanna Ambrosius Barth.

Novak, Brian H. 1991. "Alloplastic Implants for Men." *Clinics in Plastic Surgery* 18, no. 4:829–53.

Olbrisch, R. R. 1985. "Plastic and Aesthetic Surgery on Children with Down's Syndrome." *Aesthetic Plastic Surgery* 9:241–48.

Ovid. 1993. *Metamorphosen* X. Amsterdam: Athenaeum-Polak & Van Gennep.

Padmore, Catherine. 2000. "Significant Flesh: Cosmetic Surgery, Physiognomy, and the Erasure of Visual Difference(s)." *Lateral: A Journal of Textual and Cultural Studies*. www.latrobe.edu.au (last accessed March 9, 2000).

Parens, Erik. 1998a. "Is Better Always Good? The Enhancement Project." In *Enhancing Human Traits: Ethical and Social Implications*, edited by Erik Parens, 1–28. Washington, D.C.: Georgetown University Press.

———, ed. 1998b. *Enhancing Human Traits: Ethical and Social Implications*. Washington, D.C.: Georgetown University Press.

Personal Narratives Group, ed. 1989. *Interpreting Women's Lives: Feminist Theory and Personal Narratives*. Bloomington: Indiana University Press.

Phibbs, Suzanne. 2001. *Transgender Identities and Narrativity*. Ph.D. diss., University of Canterbury, New Zealand.

Piercy, Marge. 1976. *Woman on the Edge of Time*. New York: Fawcett Crest.

Piper, Adrian. 1996. "Passing for White, Passing for Black." In *Passing and the Fictions of Identity*, edited by Elaine K. Ginsberg, 234–70. Durham, N.C.: Duke University Press.

Plummer, Ken. 1983. *Documents of Life*. London: Allen & Unwin.

———. 1995. *Sexual Stories: Power, Change and Social Worlds*. London: Routledge.

Regnault, Paule. 1971. "Dr. Suzanne Noël: The First Woman To Do Esthetic Surgery." *Plastic & Reconstructive Surgery* 48, no. 2:133–39.

Reitmaier, Heidi. 1995. "'I Do Not Want to Look Like . . .': Orlan on Becoming Orlan," *Women's Art* (June 5): 5–10.

Ricoeur, Paul, with Brian Cosgrave, Gayle Freyne, David Scott, Imelda McCarthy, Redmond O'Hanlon, Brian Garvey, John Cleary, Margaret Kelleher, Dermot Moran, and Maeve Cooke. 1999. "Imagination, Testimony and Trust: A Dialogue with Paul Ricoeur." In *Questioning Ethics: Contemporary Debates in Philosophy*, edited by Richard Kearney and Mark Dooley, 12–17. London: Routledge.

Riemann, Gerhard, and Fritz Schütze. 1991. "'Trajectory' as a Basic Theoretical Concept for Analyzing Suffering and Disorderly Social Processes." In *Social Organization and Social Processes: Essays in Honor of Anselm Strauss*, edited by D. R. Maines, 333–57. New York: De Gruyter.

Rogers, Blair O. 1971. "A Chronologic History of Cosmetic Surgery." *Bulletin of the New York Academy of Medicine* 47, no. 3:265–302.

———. 1985. "The Development of Aesthetic Plastic Surgery: A History." In *The Creation of Aesthetic Plastic Surgery*, edited by Mario González-Ulloa, 1–22. New York: Springer-Verlag.

———. 1998. Foreword to *Ethnic Considerations in Facial Aesthetic Surgery*, edited by W. E. Matory Jr., xv–xviii. Philadelphia: Lippincott-Raven.

Rohrich, Rod J., and Jeffrey M. Kenkel. 1998. "The Definition of Beauty in the Northern European." In *Ethnic Considerations in Facial Aesthetic Surgery*, edited by W. Earle Matory Jr., 85–96. Philadelphia: Lippincott-Raven.

Roiphe, Katie. 1993. *The Morning After: Sex, Fear, and Feminism*. Boston: Little, Brown.

Rooks, Noliwe M. 1996. *Hair Raising: Beauty, Culture, and African American Women*. New Brunswick, N.J.: Rutgers University Press.

Russell, Kathy, Midge Wilson, and Ronald Hall. 1992. *The Color Complex: The Politics of Skin Color among African Americans*. New York: Anchor.

Saharso, Sawitri. 2003. "Culture, Toleration and Gender: A Contribution from the Netherlands." *European Journal of Women's Studies* 10, no. 1 (forthcoming).

Sarbin, Theodore, ed. 1986. *Narrative Psychology*. New York: Praeger.

Schiebinger, Londa. 1993. *Nature's Body: Gender in the Making of Modern Science*. Boston: Beacon.

Scott, Joan W. 1992. "'Experience.'" In *Feminists Theorize the Political*, edited by Judith Butler and Joan W. Scott, 22–40. New York: Routledge.

Segal, Lynne. 1990. *Slow Motion: Changing Men, Changing Masculinities*. London: Virago.

Seidler, Victor J. 1994. *Unreasonable Men: Masculinity and Social Theory*. New York: Routledge.

Shaw, George Bernard. 1916. *Pygmalion*. London: Penguin.

Shotter, John, and Kenneth Gergen, eds. 1989. *Texts of Identity*. London: Sage.

Smith, Dorothy. 1990. *Texts, Facts and Femininity: Exploring the Relations of Ruling*. London: Routledge.

Smith, Valerie. 1998. *Not Just Race, Not Just Gender*. New York: Routledge.

Stanley, Liz. 1993. *The Autobiographical I*. Manchester, U.K.: Manchester University Press.

——, ed. 1990. *Feminist Praxis: Research, Theory and Epistemology in Feminist Sociology*. London: Routledge.

Stanley, Liz, and David Morgan, eds. 1993. "Autobiography in Sociology." *Sociology* 27, no.1, special issue.

Starmans, P. M. W. 1988. "Wat gebeurt er met de esthetische chirurgie?" *Inzet: Opinieblad van de ziekenfondsen* 1:18–25.

Stepan, Nancy. 1982. *The Idea of Race in Science: Great Britain, 1800–1960*. Hamden, Conn.: Archon.

Stepan, Nancy L., and Sander L. Gilman. 1993. "Appropriating the Idioms of Science: The Rejection of Scientific Racism." In *The "Racial" Economy of Science: Toward a Democratic Future*, edited by Sandra Harding, 170–200. Bloomington: Indiana University Press.

Stephenson, Kathryn L. 1970. "The Mini-lift: An Old Wrinkle in Face Lifting." *Plastic & Reconstructive Surgery* 46, no. 3:226–35.

——. 1985. "The History of Belpharoplasty to Correct Blepharochalasis." In *The Creation of Aesthetic Plastic Surgery*, edited by Mario González-Ulloa, 23–40. New York: Springer-Verlag.

Strauss, Anselm L. 1969. *Mirrors and Masks: The Search for Identity*. Mill Valley, Calif.: Sociology Press.

Strauss, Anselm, and Barney Glaser. 1970. *Anguish: The Case Study of a Dying Trajectory*. Mill Valley, Calif.: Sociology Press.

Synnott, Anthony. 1990. "Truth and Goodness, Mirrors and Masks. Part II: A Sociology of Beauty and the Face." *British Journal of Sociology* 41, no. 1:55–76.

Taraborrelli, J. Randy. 1991. *Michael Jackson: The Magic and the Madness*. New York: Birch Lane Press.

Tate, Greg. 1992. *Flyboy in the Buttermilk: Essays on Contemporary America*. New York: Simon & Schuster.

Taylor, John. 1995. "The Long, Hard Days of Dr. Dick." *Esquire*, September.

Taylor, Paul C. 2000. "Malcolm's Conk and Danto's Colors, or, Four Logical Petitions Concerning Race, Beauty, and Aesthetics." In *Beauty Matters*, edited by Peg Zeglin Brand, 57–64. Bloomington: Indiana University Press.

Terrino, Edward O. 1991. "Implants for Male Aesthetic Surgery." *Clinics in Plastic Surgery* 18, no. 4:731–49.

Tilroe, Anna. 1996. *De huid van de kameleon. Over hedendaagse beeldende kunst.* Amsterdam: Querido.

van Dijck, José. 1995. *Manufacturing Babies and Public Consent.* London: MacMillan.

———. 1997. *Imagenation: Popular Images of Genetics.* London: MacMillan.

Wetherell, Margaret, and Nigel Edley. 1999. "Negotiating Hegemonic Masculinity: Imaginary Positions and Psycho-Discursive Practices." *Feminism & Psychology* 9, no. 3:335–56.

Wiegman, Robyn. 1995. *American Anatomies: Theorizing Race and Gender.* Durham, N.C.: Duke University Press.

Wilshire, Donna. 1989. "Uses of Myth, Image, and the Female Body." In *Gender/Body/Knowledge*, edited by Alison M. Jaggar and Susan R. Bordo, 92–114. New Brunswick, N.J.: Rutgers University Press.

Wolf, Naomi. 1991. *The Beauty Myth.* New York: Morrow.

———. 1993. *Fire with Fire.* New York: Random House.

———, ed. 1997. *Race/Sex: Their Sameness, Difference, and Interplay.* New York: Routledge.

Young, Iris Marion. 1990a. *Justice and the Politics of Difference.* Princeton, N.J.: Princeton University Press.

———. 1990b. *Throwing Like a Girl and Other Essays in Feminist Philosophy and Social Theory.* Bloomington: Indiana University Press.

Yuan, David D. 1996. "The Celebrity Freak: Michael Jackson's 'Grotesque Glory.'" In *Freakery: Cultural Spectacles of the Extraordinary Body*, edited by R. G. Thompson, 368–84. New York: New York University Press.

Zita, Jacqueline N. 1998. *Body Talk: Philosophical Reflections on Sex and Gender.* New York: Columbia University Press.

Index

facial surgery: Down's syndrome,
134–44; "face-lifts," 2, 15, 22–33,
43, 49, 51, 87, 137, 140
Featherstone, M., 118
femininity. *See* gender
feminism: 23, 36–37; and "correct
line" thinking, 15, 106, 133–34,
142; and critique of cosmetic
surgery, 3, 8–16, 35–37, 59, 73–74,
87–88, 93, 101, 103n11, 106,
110–15, 117, 129; as cultural
critique, 13–15; and women
surgeons, 15, 19–21, 23, 28, 35–37
feminist ethics, 60, 66–69
Firestone, S., 111
Flax, J., 54
Flowers, R., 123–24
Frank, A., 108
Frankford, D., 61
Fraser, N., 66. 69
Freud, S., 53–54, 107
Frosch, S., 126
Foucault, M., 6, 54–55, 74

Garfinkel, H., 74
gender: 5, 14, 28, 67, 107–09, 112–
114, 117–19, 133; and
autobiography, 52–54; and cosmetic
surgery, 3, 15, 41–44, 46–56,
125–26, 128-29, 131n10, 131n11;
femininity, 8, 10, 83–85, 88, 114,
117, 126; masculinity, 16, 52–56,
117–29; surgical ethos, of, 20,
33–37, 38n2
Gergen, K., 42, 52, 75
Gergen, M., 42, 52, 75
Giddens, A., 12–13, 18n8
Gifford, S., 124–25
Gillies, H., 31
Gilman, S., 44, 56n2, 71n5, 89–91,
102n2, 118, 130n7, 130n8, 131n9
Ginsberg, E., 90
Glaser, B., 79
González-Ulloa, M., 22, 32–33, 38n6

Gorney, M., 92
Gould, S., 90
Gubar, S., 97
Gullette, M., 118

Haiken, E., 24–25, 34, 36, 71n5, 89–91,
94, 97, 100, 118, 124, 130n8
Hall, R., 93, 102n4
Haraway, D., 6, 18n4, 109
Harding, S., 90
Hausman, B., 6, 142
Haywood, J., 28, 38n5
Hearn, J., 55
Hinderer, U., 125
Hollander, E., 30, 38n6
Hollway, W., 54
hooks, b., 93, 131n11

identity, 7, 9, 16; and biography, 42–54;
cosmetic surgery as intervention in,
73–85, 98–99, 110; inauthenticity,
140–42; racial, 96–97, 100–01;
surgeons, 46–52, 57n7;
transformation, 75–85, 96–97,
109–11. *See* "passing"
individualism, 11, 64, 119, 133
Ivy, R., 31

Jackson, M., 1, 6, 17, 88, 94–97,
99–100, 103n9
Jacobson, N., 60
Jacobus, M., 55
Jacquemin, J., 21–23, 33
Joseph, J., 33, 38n6, 44–45, 48, 89,
97–98, 102n2
justice, 92, 101, 133–34; distributive,
16, 60, 66, 68; and need
interpretation, 60, 66, 69

Kaw, E., 87, 93–94
Keller, E. F., 35, 55
Kenkel, J., 92
Klinge, I., 4
Kimmel, M., 126

About the Author

Kathy Davis is associate professor of Women's Studies in the Humanities Faculty at Utrecht University in Amsterdam, the Netherlands.